GET WELL
FOR WOMEN

A handbook of natural medicine
for women and children

GET WELL
FOR WOMEN
A handbook of natural medicine
for women and children

Russell Setright B. App. Sc., N.D., Ph. D.

Atrand Books

ATRAND Pty Ltd
Suite 2, 77 Willoughby Road
Crows Nest 2065
(02)439.5093

Bibliography
Includes index
ISBN 0 908272 28 6

1. Children—Health and hygiene—Handbooks, manuals, etc.
2. Women—Health and hygiene—Handbooks, manuals, etc.
3. Naturopathy—Handbooks, manuals, etc, I Title

615.535

Note: This book is for educational purposes only. It is not designed
to treat or diagnose disease or injuries to the body. The author, publisher
and printer accept no responsibility for such use. Never discontinue your
practitioner's medication without their advice and consult your practitioner
if suffering from any disease, injury or illness.

Printed in Australia by Griffin Paperbacks, Adelaide

THE AUTHOR
RUSSELL SETRIGHT B. App. Sc., N.D., Ph. D.
Naturopath, Herbalist and Clinician

Russell Setright is one of Australia's most well-known and leading naturopaths. His first book was the bestseller *Get Well — An A-Z of natural medicine for everyday illnesses.*

Since the 1980s he has been promoting natural therapies throughout Australia, Singapore and Malaysia on numerous radio and television shows. He writes regular newspaper and magazine columns. His current shows include a weekly talkback program on Radio 2GB, 5AA, 6PR, and 2RE, as well as regular weekly segments on various country and interstate radio stations. He has appeared on a weekly television segment on Vision TV, Toowoomba, Living in Brisbane and Good Morning Sydney. Russell is a naturopathic director at Blackmores and also has private practices at both Yagoona and Chatswood, in Sydney.

Russell Setright trained in industrial chemistry and worked in this field for 15 years and rose to the position of General Manager. Stress, poor diet, and smoking lead to a heart attack. He began studying nutrition, herbal medicine and naturopathy and restored himself to good health.

He gained a doctorate in naturopathic and traditional medicine, and a diploma of herbal medicine (with honours) in England. Russell is a Fellow of the Society of Natural Therapists and Researchers, a fellow of the Academy of Natural Therapies, a member of NHAA, ATMS, ANTA and Government Registered Naturopath (NT). He has professional qualifications in First Aid and is an instructor and examiner with St John Ambulance Australia.

Russell spends much of his weekend leisure time helping others in his position as National Flag Officer Medics in the Royal Volunteer Coastal Patrol / St John Water Ambulance and Blackmores Rescue, on a voluntary basis. He believes there is a need for more understanding between practitioners of different health care disciplines, and he is in a unique position to promote this.

ACKNOWLEDGEMENTS

There are many people I would like to thank for their help with my second book *Get Well for Women*. Firstly, my wife and family who gave me their support. To Dr S. Vij, M.B., B.S., F.R.A.C.S., F.I.C.S., from the Yagoona Medical Centre, and to Judith D'Elmaine, President of the Midwives Association, for their forewords and help. To my friend Robbie Patterson, and to Pam Tippett, for their help with the illustrations. To the Cancer Council of NSW for the use of their guide to breast examination, and to my friend Phil Daffy for his help in editing.

FOREWORD

When asked if I would write a foreword for Russell Setright's second book, *Get Well for Women*, my first thought was 'What do I know about naturopathy?' Then I thought, 'Well, I do know about women's health, particularly pregnancy, and about babies and children,' so I agreed.

Part I of the book discusses aspects of pregnancy and childbirth. It provides basic information about the beginning of life. As well, it includes signs of pregnancy with advice on how to cope with some of the discomforts which may occur in early pregnancy. There are clear drawings which show pregnant women how to do exercises which can strengthen their muscles in preparation for childbirth.

Part II of the book encompasses a compendium of information for enhancing the health of women as well as children. In Part III is a guide to the herbs used in the book. It is helpful for those who may not be familiar with what the herbs look like and their various uses.

Healthy women are the backbone of Australia. This is true not only for the contributions they make to corporate society but more importantly for the unique role they play in nurturing this country's most important resource, the future citizens, children born and unborn.

I believe that women who read this book and incorporate its principles into their daily lifestyle will be healthier, and healthy women will foster healthy children.

Judith D'Elmaine
President, NSW Midwives Association

What a joy it is for me to introduce this book to you!

I was introduced to Russell Setright through a talkback radio program one Tuesday night. The following day a patient of mine walked into my consulting room with the first edition of his book. I then acquired and read the book. It was full of useful information which is not taught in medical school or in hospital practice. Many a patient or friend approaches and asks questions and seeks information on diseases and their natural remedies. This book made me capable of answering their queries with confidence.

Herbs have been known for thousands of years and they have been helping the sick. Russell Setright is a distinguished naturopath and has been at the forefront of herbal medicine in Australia for many years.

The object of this book is to provide the interested with a straightforward practical account of natural medicines available for common ailments. The presentation is concise and clear.

I congratulate Dr Russell Setright on writing this book which will find a permanent place in many homes.

Dr S. Vij
M.B., B.S., F.R.A.C.S., F.I.C.S.

CONTENTS

Introduction

PART I
Pregnancy and childbirth   1
Having a baby   1
Early signs of pregnancy   2
Tender breasts   2
Tiredness   2
Emotions   3
Fluid retention   3
Weight gain in pregnancy   5
Carbohydrates   6
Protein   6
Fat   7
Water   7
Is there a need for supplementation with vitamins and
minerals?   7
Vitamin A and pregnancy   8
Deficiencies of vitamin A in Australian diets   10
Exercises   11
Problems during pregnancy   13
Heartburn   13
High blood pressure   13
Miscarriage   14
Morning sickness   15
Nasal congestion   15
Painful childbirth   15
Shortness of breath   16
Toxaemia   16
Eclampsia   17
The development of baby in the womb   17
The stages of labour   21
Home birth or in hospital?   22
Emergency childbirth   23
Breastfeeding   25

Vitamins and minerals in breast milk 26
Milk production 27
Cracked nipples 28
Inverted nipples 28
Cow's milk and baby 28
Allergy to cow's milk 30
Glossary of terms used in pregnancy 31

PART II
An A-Z of illnesses of women and children 34
Abrasions 34
Acne or Acne vulgaris 35
Ageing and slowing down the visible signs 36
Allergies 39
Alzheimer's Disease 43
Anaemia 46
Anal fissures 47
Anorexia nervosa and bulimia 48
Arthritis 49
Asthma 51
Athlete's foot 55
Bad breath or halitosis 57
Bedwetting 57
Birthmarks 59
Bites and stings 60
Blisters 61
Blood poisoning 62
Bloody nose (see Nosebleed)
Boils 63
Bowels (see Constipation and Diarrhoea)
Breast cancer 64
Breast self-examination 66
Bronchitis 68
Bruises 69
Bulimia (see Anorexia nervosa)
Burns 70
Candidiasis 71

Cardiovascular disease (see Immune system)
Chickenpox 72
Choking 73
Cigarette smoking 74
Cold sores (Herpes simplex) 75
Colds and flu 77
Colic 79
Concussion 79
Conjunctivitis 80
Constipation 80
Croup 82
Crying 82
Cuts and abrasions 83
Cystitis 83
Dermatitis and eczema 85
Diabetes 86
Diarrhoea 87
Dizziness 89
Dyslexia 90
Earache 91
Eczema (see Dermatitis)
Epilepsy 92
Eyes and eyesight 94
Fevers 96
Fish and fish liver oils 97
German measles (Rubella) 99
Headache 100
Heartburn (see Indigestion)
Heart disease (see Immune system, Fish oil)
Hepatitis 100
Hernia 102
Herpes (see Cold sores)
Hiccups 102
Hives 103
Hormone replacement therapy 103
Hyperactivity 105
Hypoglycaemia (Low blood sugar) 106

Hypothermia 107
Immune system and cardio vascular disease 107
Impetigo (School sores) 112
Indigestion 113
Lice 115
Menstruation 115
Motion sickness 117
Nappyrash 117
Nosebleed 118
Nutrition 118
Osteoporosis 122
Parkinson's disease 123
Shock 127
Sinusitis 128
Snoring 129
Sore throat and tonsillitis 129
Stress and vitamin B 130
Sty 132
Sunburn 133
Thrush (see Candidiasis)
Tinea (see Nappyrash)
Warts 134
Weight loss and hot foods 134

PART III
Guide to herbs used in this book 136

References 160
Index 173

INTRODUCTION

Get Well for Women is a new book and not just an update of my first book *Get Well.* The role of women and medicine is as old as time itself. We have all relied on our mothers for life, sustenance, help, care and medicine.

Being a father of four, a grandfather, and deliverer of my last child, with fifteen years of practice as a naturopath, and as a lecturer and examiner for St John Ambulance, has given me the background and materials needed to write this handbook.

Get Well for Women deals with pregnancy, childbirth, breastfeeding and babies' and children's problems, and selected problems for women of all ages such as Parkinson's disease and Hormone Replacement Therapy.

I trust you will find this book useful. It can be used in conjunction with my first book *Get Well* as a reference text in using natural medicine to promote a longer and healthier life for the whole family.

Russell Setright B. App. Sc., N.D., Ph. D.

PART I

Pregnancy and childbirth

Having a baby

Many people wait until they are financially secure before deciding to have a baby. I have found the financial security needed to afford the new arrival never comes. There is always something more to do and buy. However, all usually works out for the best.

When you decide to start a new family there are many things that need to be considered. The most important issue that needs to be addressed is nutrition, for without a balanced diet that contains all the essential vitamins and nutrients, you may not enjoy a normal healthy pregnancy and this may place baby at risk.

This may sound alarming, but the latest medical research has shown that if the mother's nutrition is inadequate, then the result could be birth defects, lower birth weight and below normal intelligence for the baby. This improvement in nutrition must start before conception, as the development of the new child begins at the moment of conception.

Diets, supplements, nutrition, birth defects and how to prevent them, will be discussed in this book under their own separate headings. Let's now discuss the changes that occur to the mother-to-be and the developing baby after conception.

After the male sperm fertilises the female egg, the egg (ovum) undergoes a change called 'cleavage' or 'cell division'. These divided cells are called blastomeres. This cell division continues to double until the embryo forms a solid mass about the size of a match head at about five weeks. At seven weeks the arms and legs have started to appear, not looking much like arms and legs but within a week they soon develop and the embryo starts looking like your new baby.

From the time of conception to full term or birth is 280 days or 10 lunar months. A lunar month is the time it takes the moon to go through a complete phase of 4 weeks. The length of the pregnancy is calculated from the first day of the last menstrual period to birth. This will give the probable date of the birth. Your practitioner may arrange an ultrasound scan during the pregnancy that will help determine a more accurate date.

Early signs of pregnancy

Tender breasts

After conception, the breasts can become very painful and sore to touch. In addition to tender breasts you will also notice an increase in the size of your breasts as they prepare for the milk needed to feed your baby. The areola (the circle of coloured skin around the nipple) becomes darker and tiny bumps all around the nipple become more prominent. At this stage you will also notice that the blood vessels in the breasts become larger. This is normal and the tenderness can be relieved by using a maternity bra for better support.

Tiredness

After conception there are enormous changes in your body as it adjusts to your growing baby. At this time it is quite normal to feel tired and run down, and some women find it hard to go about their everyday activities.

As the pregnancy progresses into the second trimester you will probably find that this is the most enjoyable time of all and easier to cope with. Feeling tired is normal and it is a sign that you need to take a rest. Don't 'overdo it'. Resting gives your body time to recuperate and adjust. Take time to put your feet up and have a little cat nap, or go to bed early. You will need all the rest you can get as after the baby arrives resting will be much more difficult.

Take your time to do your normal daily work. If you have other children, divide the work amongst them and your partner. Asking your other children to help will also make them feel needed and minimise any feelings of rejection after the birth of your baby.

Emotions

Finding out that you are pregnant can cause many different emotional effects. You may feel absolutely overwhelmed and excited. There may be times when you also may feel frightened and unable to cope. This is quite normal, preparing yourself for the responsibility of being a mother and bringing a new life into the world.

A woman may also feel that her partner will think that she is fat and unattractive. However, this is not the case. Pregnancy gives a glow and many men find that their pregnant partner is surprisingly attractive.

Fluid retention

Fluid retention during pregnancy is a problem that many mothers-to-be suffer. Quite often, when standing for long periods or in hot weather, many woman find that their ankles swell. This can be quite normal. Puffiness in the face and fingers may indicate that your kidneys are not coping with the waste products produced within your body. Also it may indicate that your placenta is not working efficiently.

It is important to drink at least 5 to 6 glasses of water per day. Cutting down on your intake of water will not help reduce fluid retention. In fact water has a diuretic effect and will help your kidneys to function well during your pregnancy. If the fluid retention is severe then discuss this with your practitioner.

SUPPLEMENTS
dandelion leaves   the leaves in salad or drink 3 cups
of dandelion tea each day

Dandelion is a non-irritating, diuretic herb that won't upset your mineral balance.

vitamin B6	one 25mg tablet with food each morning acts as a diuretic and also helps with morning sickness

Weight gain in pregnancy

During pregnancy it is normal to increase your weight by 10 to 13kg (22 to 28 pounds). Some women may put on more than this without affecting their own or the baby's health. Do not think that after the baby is born, all that is left is fat. The added weight is in the placenta, amniotic fluid, membranes and the increase in size of the breasts and uterus, combined with the increase in blood volume.

The following chart will give you the weight distribution you should expect during pregnancy.

Weight Distribution	%
your baby	38
the amniotic fluid	11
the placenta	9
increase in the breasts and uterus	20
increase in the blood	22
total weight gain	100

Baby's first kick

Feeling your baby's first movements must be one of life's most wonderful experiences, knowing that first little flutter is the sign that your baby is growing inside you. As the weeks go by the movements will get stronger and your partner will be able to experience this wonderful feeling with you. This should also make you feel more at ease, knowing that your baby is doing well and is active. By the seventh month you might see a foot shape or a little hand or bottom imprinted in your stomach.

At the end of the pregnancy before the baby's head engages, the baby will be very active, moving around from side to side. Once it has engaged, however, you will notice that the movements are much less. This is because the head is now engaged in the pelvis and is unable to move around much.

Any appreciable change in fetal activity, whether increased or decreased, may be a cause for concern and the woman should notify her medical practitioner immediately. Generally women should note 10 movements in a 12 hour period. If you don't notice any movements then contact your practitioner or the midwife.

Nutrition and pregnancy

During pregnancy it is important that all the foods that the expectant mother eats are nutritious. We are what we eat and as the developing fetus relies on the mother for nutrition, the type of foods the mother consumes could have a favourable or detrimental effect on the unborn child. It is also important that the foods the mother eats are those that will not overtax the digestive organs or organs of the eliminating systems.

Alcohol must be avoided at all costs. Clinical studies have shown that even small quantities of alcohol ingested during pregnancy could result in hyperactivity, short attention span, and emotional problems in children. Alcohol can also cause other birth deformities in the unborn baby. Alcohol fetal syndrome is thought to be caused by the mother consuming alcohol during the first three months of pregnancy (Gold S., Serry L. Hyperactivity, learning disabilities and alcohol. *Journal of Learning Disabilities*. 17(1):3-6, 1984).

Junk foods may seem nutritious but often they contain artificial colours, preservatives and flavourings. These additives are not foods and it is best to avoid them if you can.

Drugs and medications can cause problems to both mother and the fetus. Your medical practitioner or naturopath should be consulted before taking any medications. They will advise you as to their safety.

Smoking is a definite NO during pregnancy. Smoking is bad for the mother and will have an undesirable effect on the unborn fetus, such as low birth weight.

Carbohydrates

Sixty per cent of your total energy intake should be obtained from complex carbohydrates. Fresh salads, fruits and vegetables are not only nutritious but help support the organs that cleanse the blood: the kidneys and liver. These complex carbohydrate foods are high in vitamins and minerals that are essential for a healthy baby.

Don't get into the habit of only eating just one type of fruit and three types of vegetables daily. This will not give the cross-section of foods needed to supply the diet with all the micro-nutrients required. Other good sources of complex carbohydrate foods are grains including rice, wheat and corn. Potatoes are another good source of carbohydrate. Take the rainbow approach to the food on your plate. Variety is the spice of life.

Protein

Protein is the second most plentiful substance in our bodies next to water. Protein builds new tissue and repairs damaged cells. Protein is also needed for the formation of hormones and enzymes which play a variety of important functions in the body.

The building of new tissue is one of the most important roles that protein plays in the developing fetus and is therefore necessary in your diet. Eggs and dairy products are the best sources of protein, followed by meat, fish, lentils and seeds. A variety of foods containing protein should be eaten each day.

Excess protein in the diet can cause kidney damage. It is therefore important not to eat high protein foods at every meal. An example of this would be using protein drinks as a meal replacement in an endeavour to keep weight down. The energy intake from protein should be around 15 per cent of your daily diet.(See also NUTRITION in A-Z for graph on how to calculate protein).

Fat

Fats are needed in the diet as a source of the fat-soluble vitamins A, D, E and K. Fat also helps insulate our bodies and protect the unborn child and the vital organs of the body against sudden temperature changes. Fat also supplies us with the essential fatty acids that the body requires for normal metabolism. Good sources of dietary fats are fish, avocado, seeds and nuts. Meats and dairy products also are high in animal fat and cholesterol which can cause other problems.

As fat furnishes the body with twice as much energy as protein or carbohydrates, you need to eat less fat in the diet, especially if pregnant. A high fat diet will also add extra unhealthy weight to you and the unborn child. The daily intake of fat should be 25 per cent of the day's total kilojoules.

Water

This is one of the most important parts of the diet for without it the body cannot eliminate toxins that are formed by the mother and developing baby. Water helps keep the kidneys flushed and healthy.

Water can also be a source of toxic waste from our environment. I suggest that a water purifier be purchased and used to filter these toxins from the tap water before drinking. The Filter Fresh jug-type is among the best. The water is kept in the refrigerator and tastes great. Drink 6 to 8 glasses every day.

Is there a need for supplementation with vitamins and minerals ?

Many studies have shown that a lack of some vitamins and or minerals in the diet could be associated with certain types of birth defects, congenital malformations and/or spontaneous abortions.

One trial found that women who were in a high risk group of specific birth defects had a decreased incidence of birth defects including spina bifida and harelip when a multi-vitamin mineral formula was taken. (Smithhells, R. W. Spina bifida and vitamins. *British Medical Journal.* 286:388-389, 29 January 1983).

Research has also shown that the diets of pregnant women in Australia and the USA (as in many other parts of the world) are low in blood zinc levels. A report in the *American Journal of Clinical Nutrition.* 40: 496-507, 1984 found that women who had low plasma zinc levels had more complications of pregnancy, including maternal infections and fetal distress. Other reports stated that the recommended dietary intake could not easily be obtained through diet alone. Brewer's yeast, eggs, and wheat germ are all good sources of zinc. There are many parts of the world, in particular Australia, New Zealand and the USA, where the zinc levels in the soil are poor.

Folic acid   During pregnancy the requirements for folic acid double. Good food sources are egg yolks, pumpkins, deep green vegetables and brewer's yeast.

Calcium   The need for calcium by the mother and developing baby also doubles during pregnancy. Good food sources are dairy products, blackstrap molasses and sesame seeds.

Recommended supplementation.

Naturetime Multi-vitamin mineral formula (sustained release)	1 tablet morning with food
calcium	1,000mg to 1,500mg daily
folic acid	0.8mg daily during pregnancy
red raspberry leaf tea	drink 3 cups daily during the third trimester
evening primrose oil	500iu 3 times daily
iron phosphate	15mg 3 times daily
magnesium phosphate	500mg daily

Vitamin A and pregnancy

Vitamin A is a fat-soluble vitamin that occurs in nature in two forms: preformed vitamin A which is only found in certain tissues of animals, mainly the liver, and beta-carotene. This preformed vitamin A is metabolised by animals from carotene (pro-vitamin A) in their food.

Vitamin A helps build resistance to infection and supports the integrity of the mucous membranes of the respiratory, urinary and digestive tracts. Vitamin A is also essential for the normal growth of strong bones and teeth in children and is necessary for fertility in both men and women.

It must be understood that many of the foods we eat each day contain vitamin A, and providing we eat sensibly, these foods are very safe.

Expectant mothers however should not eat large quantities of vitamin A rich foods, foods contributing more than 25,000iu of vitamin A to the daily diet.

crab	9,800iu per 453g
liver	8,000 -10,000iu per 100g(3.5oz)
halibut	2,000iu per 100g
fresh salmon	1,359iu per 100g
liverwurst	28,800iu per 100g
butter	7,500iu per cup
cod liver oil	5,000iu per teaspoon approx.
milk	350iu per cup
cheddar cheese	1,197iu per cup
human breast milk	560iu per cup approx.

human colostrum around twice that of breast milk

SUPPLEMENTS

In Australia the recommended dietary intake (RDI) of vitamin A as retinol equivalents (RE) needed to maintain normal body functions in a healthy individual is:

babies — birth to 6 months	300 mcg = 1,000iu
babies — 6 months to 1 year	450 mcg = 1,498iu
1 year to 5 years	300 mcg = 1,000iu
6 years to 8 years	400 mcg = 1,332iu
12 years to 15 years	725 mcg = 2,420iu
15 years and over	750 mcg = 2,500iu

Vitamin A is vital for the healthy development of the unborn child. During pregnancy the RDI is 2,500iu of vitamin A which must be obtained from the diet or by supplementation each day. When breastfeeding, the RDI increases to 4,000iu daily.

There is evidence that the excessive intake of vitamin A in pregnancy may lead to birth defects. Some medical researchers state that pregnant woman should avoid vitamin A (retinol) in amounts over 25,000iu daily.

It is very important if expecting a child not to eat large quantities of liver and meat offal as these contain very high levels of vitamin A. If taking a vitamin A supplement then always follow the directions. Research has shown that some women, especially those women born in the United Kingdom, may be consuming levels as high as 283,050iu per day. These high intakes could lead to birth defects, therefore organ offal meats as part of the diet should be avoided.

Under medical supervision, doses of up to 50,000iu of vitamin A (retinol) are used for severe deficiency in children over 8 years of age and adults. Vitamin A has also been used therapeutically in doses of up 300,000iu daily for five months with minimum side effects for the treatment of acne vulgaris. However, these amounts of vitamin A should not be consumed during pregnancy.

Deficiencies of vitamin A in Australian diets

The Department of Community Services and Health commissioned two reports: the National Dietary Survey of Adults (1983) and the National Dietary Survey of Schoolchildren from 10 to 15 years of age (1985).

These reports found that up to 62 per cent of girls aged between 10 and 15 years, and 49 per cent of boys in the same age group were receiving less than the RDI (recommended dietary intakes) of REs (retinol equivalents). The reports also found that up to 50 per cent of women aged between 25 years and 64 years, and up to 42 per cent of men in the same age group were receiving less than the RDI of retinol equivalents.

Exercises

As you prepare for the birth of your child you will need to do exercises to be in peak condition for the experience. The following are simple and undemanding. Do not do any strenuous lifting or exercising during the pregnancy.

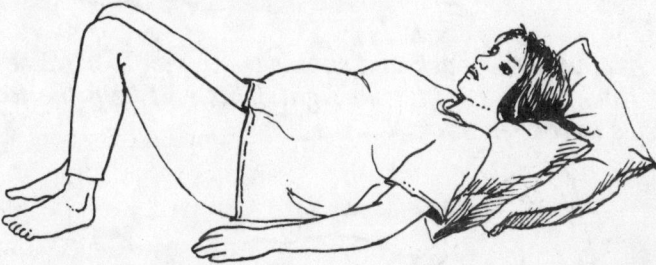

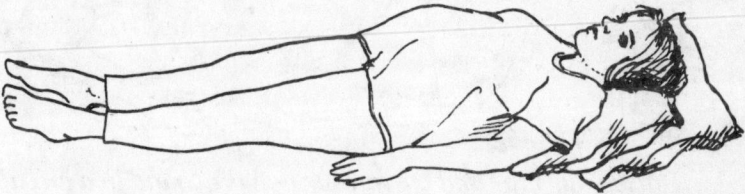

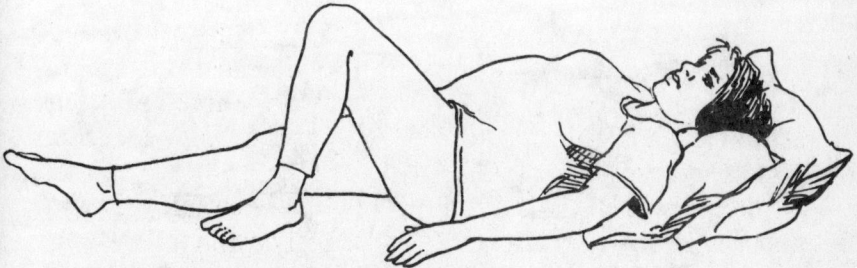

Lie on the floor with a pillow under your head. Raise your knees and press the small of your back to the floor. Slowly extend your legs until they are both straight. Lift one leg then the other, while your back remains on the floor. This exercise tones up the stomach muscles.

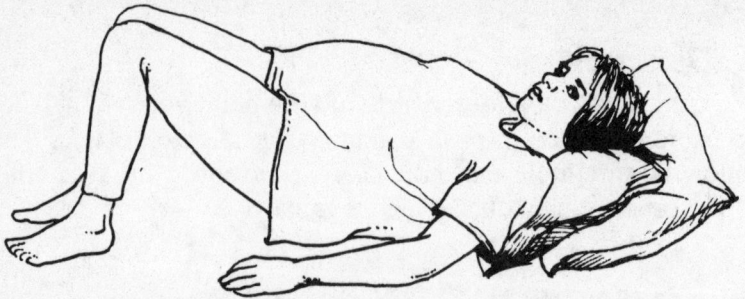

Keeping your back and shoulders to the floor, raise your hips. Rock them from left to right. This will help the tone of muscles in your buttocks.

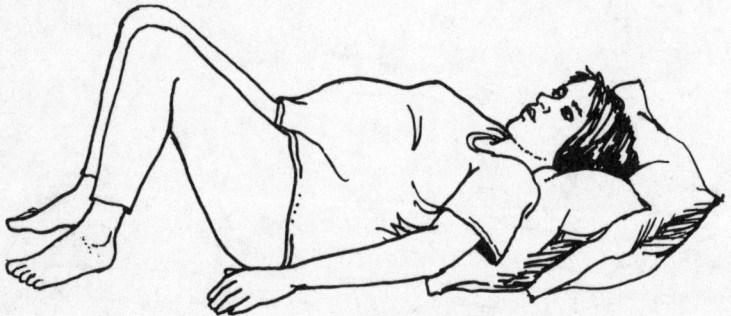

Raise your hips and move your pelvis around in a circular motion to help strengthen pelvic muscles.

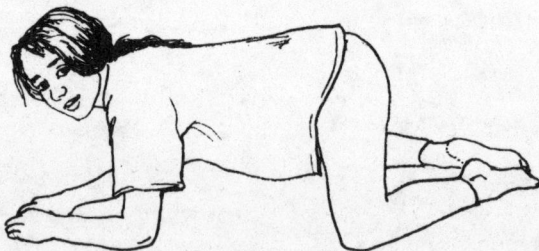

Get on your knees and elbows and make your back flat, not sagging in the middle. Push your back up to a 'cat's arch' and then bring it down to the flat position again. This strengthens the spine and relieves lower backache.

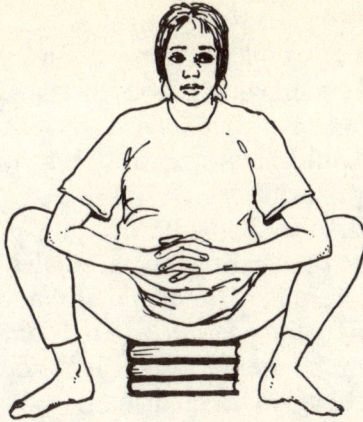

Squatting on a stool or a pile of books relieves backache and opens the pelvis.

Problems during pregnancy

Heartburn

Heartburn and indigestion can be a common and uncomfortable complaint in the last three or four months of pregnancy. Heartburn is a result of the stomach acids flowing back into the oesophagus causing the burning and uncomfortable pain.

To help reduce the pressure on the stomach, eat smaller meals, say five small meals daily instead of the normal three. Also, fatty and spicy foods can aggravate the problem. Ensure that your clothes are not too tight around the stomach and when sitting, or in bed, use a pillow to help make yourself comfortable, as this will ease the problem.

The herbs slippery elm and peppermint taken in combination will quickly bring relief. Acid-Eze contains these and a teaspoon three times a day is recommended.

High blood pressure

High blood pressure is a dangerous condition at any time and if you suspect that you may be suffering from this condition, then you should discuss this with your practitioner.

Your weight and the foods you eat play an important role in the prevention of hypertension. It is therefore very important to maintain the correct weight-for-term during your pregnancy. Celery, apples and cucumber are foods that have natural diuretic properties so they are also good foods to pick on when you have a craving for something that may not be as nutritious. These foods are also low in calories.

Supplementing the diet with evening primrose oil and calcium can also be of benefit. Clinical studies have found that by supplementing the diet of women with evening primrose oil and/or calcium their blood pressure was reduced. One trial found that supplementing the diet of pregnant women with between 1,000mg and 2,000mg of calcium daily reduced their blood pressure, and may prevent the onset of pregnancy induced hypertension, (Kawasaki, N. et al. Effect of calcium supplementation on the vascular sensitivity to angotensin 11 in pregnant women. *American Journal of Obstetrics and Gynaecology* 153(5):576-82, 1985).

Supplementation with evening primrose oil may also help slow the development of, or prevent, high blood pressure during pregnancy. I have found that evening primrose oil, at a dose of one to two 500mg capsules up to three times daily, effectively treats hypertension.

Miscarriage

When the fetus is developing in the early stages, there is always the possibility of miscarriage or abortion. Sometimes this is not noticed by the mother-to-be as the developing fetus may miscarry at the time of the next period which may be just a little heavier than normal.

Vitamin E may prevent miscarriage. There is reasonable evidence that vitamin E may prevent habitual or recurring miscarriages. Vitamin E given to expectant mothers who had a history of miscarriages has been shown to reduce the incidence of miscarriage (Sutton, R.V. Vitamin E in habitual abortion, *British Medical Journal.* 858, 4 October 1958). Do not eat potatoes if they have any green spots as they may contain solanine. This is a poisonous narcotic alkaloid that can cause miscarriage.

Morning sickness

There is some evidence that vitamin B6 (pyridoxine) may help relieve the symptoms of morning sickness. The symptoms of morning sickness can include nausea and vomiting. Usually the amount of vitamin B6 contained in a good multi vitamin and mineral formula is sufficient to help relieve these symptoms. However, high doses of this vitamin should be avoided late in pregnancy as studies have shown that high doses of vitamin B6 may shut off breast milk. It must therefore be reduced before delivery in mothers who plan to breastfeed their new babies.

I have found that peppermint tea is helpful in relieving the symptoms of morning sickness. Drink one cup of peppermint tea and eat a piece of toast before getting out of bed in the morning and two more cups during the day. This will need the help of the father-to-be in the morning and he should remember that his duty to the unborn child started with conception. Another herb that I have found relieves morning sickness symptoms is ginger. Travel Calm Ginger is recommended. Take one tablet every 4 hours.

Nasal congestion

Often in pregnancy the mucous membranes inside the nostrils and sinuses swell and the symptoms of a head cold may be there all the time. This congestion is the result of the increase in blood volume and the changes in your hormones. Although breathing through your nose may be more difficult, it will not interfere with your labour.

A little eucalyptus and camphor on your pillow at night or a vaporiser in the room can often help. Cow's milk can also be mucous forming and may aggravate the problem. Use soy milk instead.

Painful childbirth

Raspberry leaf has been used for hundreds of years for helping relieve the pain of childbirth . This herb has the ability to relax the smooth muscle of the uterus, making raspberry leaf useful as an aid to parturition (Burn, J.H. A principle in raspberry leaves which relaxes uterine muscles. *Lancet.* 2 (6149) 1-3, 1941). Drink one cup of raspberry leaf tea three times daily during the third trimester.

Shortness of breath

When you reach about 34 weeks and your baby is high in the womb, pressure will be placed on the diaphragm which may be moved out of place as much as 2.5cm (1 inch). This in turn can cause shortness of breath. Even bending over can be very exhausting. Sleeping propped up, or when sitting, placing a pillow behind your back, will help enormously. Shortness of breath is also a reminder of the need to take things easy, slow down and have a well deserved rest.

Toxaemia

Toxaemia is not a word which is currently used. Today, the word pre-eclampsia is used and relates to a condition in which the blood pressure is raised and there may be associated swelling of the hands and face as well as the feet and ankles. Protein may also be passed in the urine. Toxaemia is a serious problem that can affect women during pregnancy. There is an added strain on the mother's kidneys and liver during pregnancy. Not only do these organs need to eliminate the toxins that are produced by the mother but they must also remove all waste products and toxins that are produced by the developing fetus. Other toxins that may be produced are also absorbed into the mother's blood stream. If these toxins build up in the mother's blood and the eliminatory organs are unable to remove them, then a condition known as toxaemia may result.

If the expectant mother has a history of high blood pressure or kidney disease it is important that she advise her practitioner as this may lead to complications later in the pregnancy.

Symptoms that should be reported to your practitioner are: swelling of the feet and legs, high blood pressure, puffiness of the face and/or severe headaches or dizziness and any increase in your temperature.

Any or all of these symptoms could indicate a problem that needs professional advice and treatment.

Eclampsia

This is fitting which can occur when 'toxaemia' is unable to be controlled. This is a major toxaemia of pregnancy and is accompanied by high blood pressure. Eclampsia most often affects the kidney, liver, brain and placenta. This is a very serious condition and must be managed in hospital. The life of the mother and the unborn child could be placed at risk if time is wasted.

The development of your baby in the womb

First Month By the third or fourth week, or end of the first lunar month the heart, head, eyes and backbone are formed. In a primitive form, the digestive, urinary and circulatory systems appear.

Second Month The embryo continues to develop and by the second month of the pregnancy the toes begin to separate, the fingers and eyelids are formed. The newly developing baby has already taken the shape and physical looks of a child. At this stage the embryo is still only 2.5 cm (1 inch) long.

Third Month In the third month (12 weeks) the face, limbs, arms and neck are more perfectly formed. The nails on the fingers and toes begin to appear and the first signs of the sex of the developing embryo now begin to show. Baby is now about 6.5 cm (2.5 inches) in length.

Fourth Month As mother and child enter the fourth month of pregnancy the placenta, or afterbirth, begins to play an important role. This placenta (a configuration of blood vessels surrounding the fetus) supplies oxygen and nutrients to the fetus. These nutrients are taken from the blood of the mother and at the same time the placenta detoxifies the fetal blood, removing impurities from the fetus and returning them to the mother's blood stream for excretion by the mother's organs (kidneys, lungs, intestines and skin).

Now the first signs of hair on the fetus begin to appear on the head and other parts of the body. The developing fetus is now approximately 8-9 cm (3.5 inches) in length.

Fifth Month Baby is now entering the fifth month and mother can now feel the baby start to move. This is one of the most exciting times for the new parents as the realisation that the swollen tummy and clothes that don't fit any more forecast a new life.

During this month, your practitioner can hear the sounds of the baby's heart for the first time. This is very exciting and the parents should ask their practitioner if they could listen. This will help develop a special closeness and love.

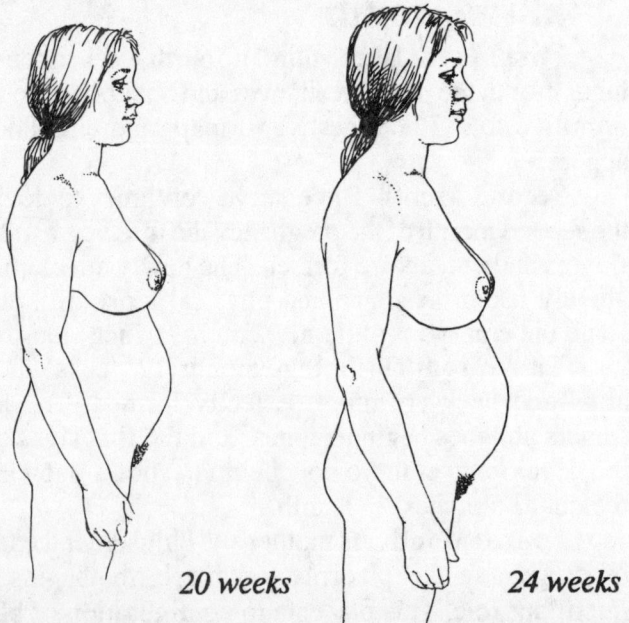

20 weeks *24 weeks*

Sixth Month As mother and the unborn child enter the sixth month the hair is starting to grow longer and the eyelashes and eyebrows are now formed. If baby is born at this time it could live but the lungs are not yet fully formed and the fetus might die. Modern medicine has, however, made great advances in the treatment and management of premature infants and the chances now for survival are improving all the time. Baby now weighs about 0.5 kg (1.10 pounds) and is approximately 32 cm (13 inches) in length.

Seventh Month Mother and the unborn child are now entering the seventh month (28 weeks). Baby could weigh as much as 0.9 kgs (2 pounds) and have attained a length of 38 cm (14.5 inches). The nails now break through the thin covering that protects them and the membrane that has covered the eyes over the past six months starts to disappear. As body fat increases the skin starts to smooth out and the unborn child resembles a full term child. If baby is born at this time then the chances of survival are much better.

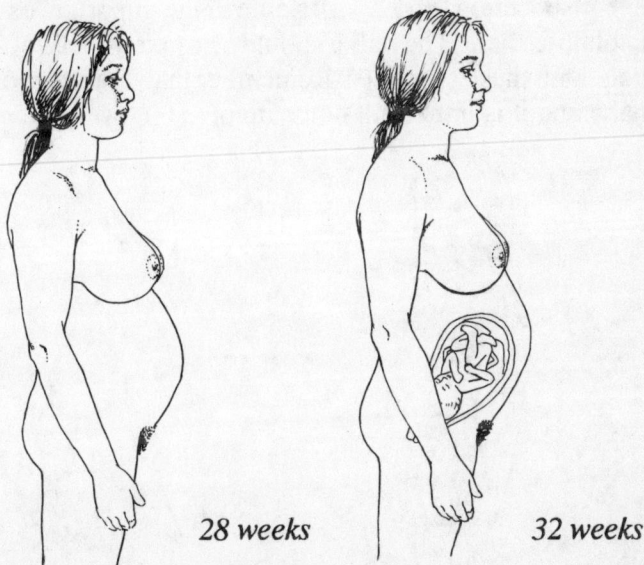

28 weeks   *32 weeks*

Eight Month In the eighth month (32 weeks) the fetal weight increases along with length. Baby is now approaching 42 cm (16 inches) in length. Kicking and movement can be felt and the father usually receives a number of kicks from the baby in bed. A foot or arm can also be seen pushing against the mother's stomach from time to time. This is another exciting time as the parents realise more fully that in a few weeks a new life will arrive.

Ninth Month The ninth month (36 weeks) arrives, and it is at this time the mother feels the most uncomfortable, as it is during this month that the fetus moves into position in readiness for the birth. The fine hair that covered the entire body of the fetus has almost gone and the nails have reached the end of the fingers and toes. The unborn child's head bones are soft and easily moulded into the shape of the mother's pelvis. Baby's weight is now approximately 2.7 kg (5.5 pounds) with a length of 49 cm (18 inches).

The exercises that have been learned during the prenatal classes now become more difficult. It is important to keep them up. For those who did not attend prenatal classes, turn to the exercise section (pp 11-13). Some of the important exercises are explained there. The father should also take an active interest and help with these exercises. Remember that it takes two to make a baby and it is important he be involved in everything.

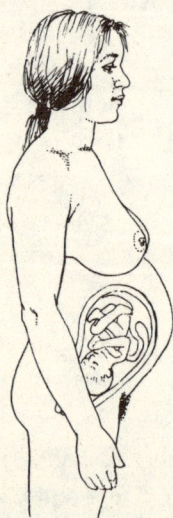 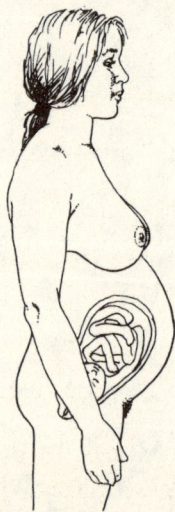

36 weeks   *40 weeks*

Full term Finally the tenth month (40 weeks), full term and the baby is fully developed and ready to enter the world. This is the time when the suitcases are packed and everybody jumps at the first sign of any pains. Baby is now approximately 55 cm (21.5 inches) in length.

The stages of labour

Some women experience pains similar to labour pains from the seventh month onwards. These pains are known as 'false labour pains'. If you have these pains, and they last a long time or are associated with a show of blood or water, then see your practitioner or go to the nearest hospital.

First stage

True labour pains occur in the lower abdomen and are cramp-like in nature. These pains usually last from 15 to 30 seconds and are spaced 10 to 20 minutes apart. When these pains start then the mother is in the first stage of labour.

It is common to have a 'show', a 'show' being the term used to describe the bloodstained mucous. This is followed later, especially after a labour pain, by water. This is known as the breaking of the waters. The waters, or liquor amnii, are produced by the thin lining membrane called 'the amnion'. This fluid encases the unborn baby, protecting it from external harm. The waters are also important as they lubricate and cleanse the birth canal and help dilate the cervix.

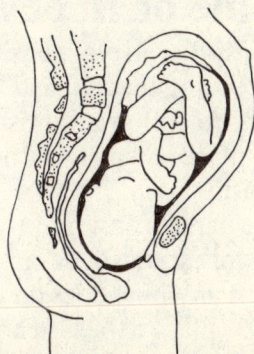

Second stage

The second stage of labour is said to have started when the cervix is fully dilated (expanded). In this stage the contractions will occur every two to three minutes, they may even be more frequent and usually last one to two minutes.

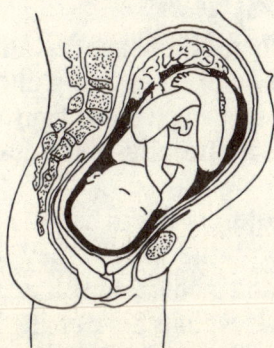

Undilated cervix   *Dilated cervix*

The mother will now have a desire to bear down or push and at this stage she should be encouraged to pant, keeping her mouth open and not holding her breath.

There will be a bulging of the perineum and an increase in the flow of the bloodstained waters. Baby's head should now be visible and be facing the mother's anus. As the birth progresses the baby's head will usually turn to one side.

With the next push, if all is going to plan, the most exciting experience occurs, the birth of the new baby. This newcomer to our world is wet and slippery and is still attached to the mother by the umbilical cord.

Third stage

The third stage of labour is the delivery of the placenta or afterbirth, up to 10 or more minutes after the birth of the baby. To encourage the expulsion of the placenta, the baby will be put on the mother's breast. This breastfeeding will also help the uterus to contract and control bleeding.

The new child

The wonder of the creation of this new life will last a lifetime. Parents and relatives, after counting all the fingers and toes, are already looking closely at the baby's ears, nose, and chin to decide which members of the family the baby takes after.

Home birth or in hospital?

As with all well planned events, there is a chance that all will not go according to plan, and the arrival of a new baby into the world is no exception to this rule. Babies can be born at any time and at any place and this may not be near a hospital or the desired place of birth.

Some parents now, as in days of old, choose to have a home birth in familiar surroundings and with the people they love. However, if anything does go wrong and medical help is needed then the best place to be is in hospital. Hospitals have changed in their attitudes to family involvement in the birth of a baby over the past years. The image of the father sitting in a little room out the back smoking cigarettes while the expectant mother lies in an unfriendly room, is no longer true. The truth is that many hospitals encourage the father-to-be by the mother's side and play an active part in the joyous event. I have found that midwives are not only expert in what they do but also give helpful and loving emotional support. Also most hospitals allow the father and/or close relatives to visit the new mum and baby whenever they like. However, if a home birth is decided upon then it is important to have a qualified midwife in attendance because during the birth of a baby, although it is a natural and usually uncomplicated event, things can go wrong. A friendly hospital may be your best choice.

Emergency childbirth

If the situation arises that you are unable to get to hospital and the birth of your new baby is imminent then it is important to have an idea what to do. I would suggest that you talk to your practitioner about this during your pregnancy.

If the pains are bearing down in nature and/or the waters have broken then the birth may be imminent and you should prepare for the birth. The following is a guide on how to deliver a baby in an emergency.

Call for an ambulance or medical aid

Then wash your hands and arms using soap, a nail brush and hot water.

You will need the following:

1. Three clean sheets
2. A sharp pair of sterilised scissors to cut the umbilical cord
3. Three lengths of string or cotton tape that have been boiled for a minimum of 10 minutes
4. Clean towels
5. Dettol or other antiseptic
6. Some nappies to wrap baby in

7. A light blanket to keep the mother warm after the birth
8. A clean handkerchief or face mask
9. Sterile cotton wool swabs

Preparing the delivery bed

The expectant mum will need a suitable place to lie. Prepare this using a clean sheet if possible, then under the mother starting from the waist, cover the sheet with plastic and extend all the way to the end of the sheet. A new, clean, opened up garbage bag will do. This should then be covered with an absorbent material. A few layers of opened up newspaper will suffice if you don't have anything sterile. This must then be covered with another clean sheet. Wash your hands again and allow to air-dry.

The mother should be placed on the prepared bed with the lower half of her body over the sheet covering the plastic area. She should be on her back with her knees drawn up. With each contraction she will want to push. The mother must be encouraged at this time to pant with her mouth open and not to hold her breath, and to bear down.

When the baby's head first appears, apply firm but gentle pressure in a backwards and slightly upwards direction. This will help prevent the baby being born too quickly. As the head appears it should be facing down and will slowly turn to one side during the birth. The head needs to be supported and controlled through the whole delivery.

At this stage it can be seen if the umbilical cord is around the baby's neck. If it is, then gently pull the loop of the umbilical cord over the baby's head. If this cannot be carried out, then try to loosen the cord enough to allow the baby to pass through the loop at birth.

The next contraction should deliver the baby's shoulders. Once the shoulders are born, then the rest of the baby will follow on the next contraction. In preparation for this, and during the next contraction, support the baby under the armpits and lift upwards towards mother's abdomen. The baby is now born.

Baby will be covered with mucous and be very slippery.

Taking care, wrap the baby in a clean towel or nappy. With one hand hold both ankles. One ankle should be held between the index finger and the thumb. The other three fingers fold around the other ankle.

Baby should now be held upside down. Your other hand should be supporting the head and neck. This allows the fluid to drain from the airways (throat, nose and mouth). Use the cotton wool swabs to wipe away the blood and mucous from the baby's nose, mouth and eyes. Remember that the umbilical cord is still attached to the placenta within the mother. Do not try to pull the cord out.

When the baby cries place it on the mother's abdomen to nurse. The baby should be encouraged to suckle the breast. This will help in expelling the afterbirth: the third stage of labour.

Following the expulsion of the placenta, the umbilical cord can be cut, but only after it has stopped pulsating.

You will now need the three pieces of sterile string or tape and the scissors. Tie the first tape around the cord 10 cms (4 inches) from the baby's navel. It is important that these tapes be tied firmly as failure to do so could result in the newborn baby bleeding from the cord. The next tie is located 15 cms (6 inches) from the navel and the third tie should be 20 cms (8 inches) from the navel. The cord may now be cut between the second and third ties; these are the ties farthest away from the baby.

The mother can now be washed and a sanitary napkin placed in position. Remember to retain the sanitary napkin and placenta for inspection by her practitioner. A cup of peppermint or chamomile tea and a rest are recommended.

Breastfeeding

There is no entirely satisfactory substitute for breast milk. When it comes to feeding baby, breast is best.

Breast milk not only contains all the important nutrients, water ratio, vitamins and minerals that baby needs, it also comes in a container ready to use and does not need heating in the middle of the night. Mother's milk is always at the right temperature and is free.

Colostrum, or first milk, is a mixture of mainly serum and white blood cells transferred from the mother. Colostrum continues to flow in small amounts, before the start of true lactation, for the first two or three days after birth.

One of the reasons that the colostrum precedes the normal breast milk is that it transfers part of the mother's immunity to the baby. This gives baby a good start and it is very important that, even if you have decided not to breastfeed your baby in the future, at least the first few days of baby's nourishment should be supplied by the mother.

The main reason for not breastfeeding, given by many mothers, is financial. Many situations require the mother to start work again soon after the birth of her baby and therefore breastfeeding becomes impractical. Others include an inability to feed the baby due to poor breast milk quality or quantity and this may be due to one or more problems, including stress. Your practitioner, midwife or the Nursing Mothers' Association may be able to solve your problem.

If one of the reasons you decide to discontinue breastfeeding is a lack of breast milk then there are many things that can be done to help. Unfortunately the stressful lifestyles that many of us lead can prevent the mother from relaxing. It is best to avoid excitement and worry. This is very important as relaxation helps 'let down', the term used to describe the flow of milk, into the breasts ready for baby to feed.

Incorrect stimulation of the nipples by the baby can be caused by incorrect positioning of the baby during feeding. This positioning will prevent the baby sufficiently stimulating the nerves in the nipples resulting in a reduced flow of breast milk. Incorrect positioning of the baby during feeding can also cause the nipples to become painful as baby will pull on the nipple to receive the amount of milk required. The best position for baby when feeding is chest to chest and chin to breast.

Vitamins and minerals in breast milk

Although breast milk is almost perfect food it may be low in vitamin C, iron and vitamin D. It is recommended to supplement the mother's diet with these nutrients in order for baby to receive adequate quantities of these substances in the breast milk. Blackcurrant juice is one of the best sources of vitamin C. Ribena is a vitamin C formula based on blackcurrants.

During lactation it is imperative that mother's nutrition is maintained, as poor nutrition will alter the quality of the breast milk. If good nutrition is not maintained then the mother's body will be robbed of vital nutrients as it endeavours to maintain the quality of the breast milk.

It is not unusual for a mother to lose the enamel from her teeth, or to start to lose hair, while lactating. This is usually related to poor nutrition. Remember that the loss of blood during birth reduces the mother's nutrients, including iron, and these need to be replaced.

Mother should include brewer's yeast, whole grain cereals, eggs, milk and meats in the diet. These foods are rich in many of the extra nutrients that are required during lactation. Also, eat fresh fruits and vegetables every day as these are a must.

Unless mother is eating lots of dairy products then she will need to supplement her diet with extra calcium phosphate. Calcium phosphate is needed to prevent bone loss and teeth deterioration and this nutrient is even more important during nursing than in pregnancy.

Milk production

In combination with a well-balanced diet there are many herbs to improve the production of breast milk. These include aniseed, goat's rue, fennel seeds and caraway seeds that can all be made into teas.

Goat's rue (*Galega officinalis*) is the strongest of these herbs. Three cups of the tea made from two tablespoons of the herb in one cup of boiling water may be taken safely each day to help increase the flow of milk.

Another refreshing drink can be made by mixing 1 part of aniseed (*Pimpinella anisum*), 1 part of fenugreek seeds (*Trigonella foenum-graecum*) and 1 part of fennel seeds (*Foeniculum vulgare*). The seeds will need to be crushed, added to cold water and slowly brought to the boil and simmered for 10 minutes. Add the aniseed and stand for 10 minutes, filter and drink 1 cup 3 times daily.

To supplement the loss of minerals, take one tablet daily of Naturetime multi vitamin and mineral formula. A calcium phosphate formula containing 800 to 1,500mg of calcium is recommended daily.

Cracked nipples

Prevention is the best policy. Exposure to natural sunlight and fresh air can help prevent cracked and sore nipples. A few minutes in the morning sun will help. Nursing pads should also be replaced when they become wet. If in-between leakage is a problem then use a little ice cold water on and around the nipple area. This will help prevent this problem.

A mixture of wool fat (lanolin) and Friar's Balsam lightly applied to cracked nipples will usually solve the problem. It may sting a little but it is very healing. Vitamins A, B and C will also help prevent cracking of the nipples.

Inverted nipples

Dr Lady Cilento suggested the use of a Woolwich nipple shield (available from chemists) to help overcome the problem. Manipulating the nipple between the fingers will stimulate the erectile tissue in the nipple. Pull the nipple out and massage regularly. This will help the nipple stand out and will assist in the breastfeeding process.

Cow's milk and baby

Many mothers unfortunately believe that cow's milk is as good as breast milk once baby has received the colostrum or once mother and baby are home from hospital. This is not the case as there are so many differences between cow's milk and mother's milk that make cow's milk an unacceptable food for baby.

The chart shows the difference between the two milks.

Constituents	Cow's milk	Mother's milk
	%	%
protein	3 - 4	1.5l
lactose (milk sugar)	4.5	7.0
fat	3.5	3.5
mineral salts	0.6	0.2
water	87.4 - 88.4	87.8
TOTAL	100.0	100.0

Another difference is that mother's milk is alkaline and cow's milk is slightly acid. Although this is not a major problem it needs to be considered.

If you decide to use cow's milk to feed baby then it must be modified. Talk this over with your clinic sister or practitioner. The usual method used is to dilute the cow's milk with 50 per cent boiled water. This reduces the protein content of the milk to around that of mother's milk. This dilution also reduces the carbohydrate (milk sugar). The addition of sugar of milk or lactose will solve this problem. As the fat content of this formula is less than that of human breast milk, add cod liver oil emulsion to the formula. Cod liver oil is a good source of both vitamin A and D. Dr Lady Cilento and Sister Kenny recommended cod liver oil as a vitamin and fatty acid supplement for babies.

Cod liver oil dosage: place a few drops on the back of the baby's tongue daily. Increase to 4mls (a little less than a teaspoon) each day by 12 months. Babies thrive on it.

Mixing instructions for 600ml of baby's formula

cow's or goat's milk	300ml
boiled water	300ml
lactose (sugar of milk)	2 tablespoons
cod liver oil emulsion	1 tablespoon

A better way of feeding baby if you cannot breastfeed would be to use a commercially prepared formula. There are many different types of formula available, usually based on a modified cow's milk formula or using soy bean milk. My preference if breastfeeding baby is not the chosen method would be a formula based on soy bean milk protein. The protein of soy beans is alkaline and is more easily digested by baby. Unlike cow's milk, soy milk formulas are also less liable to cause any adverse reactions such as milk allergy.

It is important to remember that commercially available formulas don't contain the mother's antibodies or enzymes as does breast milk, and they are not breast milk in a can.

Allergy to cow's milk

True allergy to cow's milk results from the infant having a reaction to the protein of cow's milk. This reaction can include asthma, eczema, loose motions, thrush and colic. Many people confuse cow's milk allergy with lactose intolerance which is caused by an ability of the baby to digest the lactose in milk. This inability to digest lactose is a result of a deficiency of the enzyme lactase, an enzyme that is normally found in the intestine. Without this enzyme, lactose cannot be broken down and absorbed into the blood stream of the baby. The lactose that is in the intestine is seen by the body as a foreign substance and is flushed from the intestines, causing diarrhoea.

If you suspect that your child has an allergy to cow's milk then try using either goat's milk or soy bean milk. If the problem is one of lactose intolerance then a formula free of lactose will be needed; 20 per cent of children who have a lactose intolerance may also have an intolerance to sucrose. It is best to choose a formula that contains neither lactose nor sucrose.

Most of these problems can be avoided by breastfeeding as long as possible.

Glossary of terms used in pregnancy

abdomen	stomach/belly area
afterbirth	the placenta
amniotic fluid	the liquid the baby floats in, the waters
amniotic sac	the bag holding the waters and baby
Apgar scale	tests carried out on the newborn baby
birth canal	the vagina
cervix	the neck of the womb
conception	the union of the male sperm and the female egg (ovum); fertilisation
contractions	a tightening of the womb muscle
EDC	expected date of confinement
egg	the ovum or female cell
embryo	the ball of cells formed in the first weeks of pregnancy
fallopian tubes	the tubes that lead from the ovary to the womb

fertilisation	conception, the union of the male and female cells
fetus	the name given to the baby after 12 weeks
hormone	a chemical which controls part of the body's function
internal examination	your medical practitioner will insert one or two fingers into the vagina to determine if all is going to plan
navel	the belly button
ovary	the female organ that produces the egg
ovum	the female cell or egg
placenta	the afterbirth
prenatal exercises	exercises for mothers-to-be
quickening	the baby's first movements that are felt by the mother
sperm	the male cell in the fluid ejected from the penis
term	the time from the 37th week of pregnancy to the birth or 42nd week

tubes	the fallopian tubes
umbilical cord	the cord of tissue and blood vessels that connect the placenta to the baby's navel
uterus	the womb
vagina	the birth canal
womb	the uterus

PART II

An A—Z of illnesses of women and children

Abrasions

Abrasions are usually very painful and if not properly attended to can leave a scar. Abrasions are one of the most common injuries that children have. An abrasion is a break or cut in the skin that is wider and longer than it is deep, and not full skin thickness but shallow.

The wound must be cleaned properly. Soap and water is best. Wash the abrasion along the length of the wound so that all the imbedded dirt is removed. Use an antiseptic on the area to prevent infection. Tea tree oil is effective. Add a little tea tree oil to a moist cotton wool ball and gently dab the area of the wound. Cover the area with a sterile non-stick dressing and lightly bandage.

When a scab forms it must not be picked off as this will only cause scarring and may also reinfect the wound. At this stage use a Healing Ointment based on comfrey, vitamin A, and vitamin E. This will help speed up the healing process and keep the scab supple.

As the healing process requires vitamins and minerals to help the body form new skin and heal quickly, ensure your child's diet includes plenty of fresh fruits, vegetables and whole grains. These are good sources of vitamin C and zinc; these nutrients help form collagen (the skin cement), fight infection and help prevent scarring.

Supplementing the child's diet with a children's multi-vitamin and mineral formula will ensure that they are receiving all the vitamins and minerals lacking in the diet. If infection cannot be controlled, or your child develops a fever, consult your practitioner.

TOPICAL TREATMENT

Tea tree oil	apply twice daily on the first day or if infection is still present
Healingand Golden Seal Ointments	apply to the scab and new forming skin areas twice daily

SUPPLEMENTS

children's multi-vitamin and mineral formula	1 tablet daily

Acne or *Acne vulgaris*

Acne vulgaris is most commonly caused by the hormonal changes of adolescence. Adolescent girls produce more of the hormone oestrogen and boys, androgen. These hormones lead to an increase in the activity of the sebaceous glands of the skin on the face, neck and back. Sebum, the sticky substance produced by these glands, can fill the skin pores resulting in blackheads and whiteheads. If these become blocked and infected the skin becomes inflamed and covered with red and purplish pimples which may disappear, or in more extreme cases, cause scarring. For the adolescent who has a new and sudden interest in body image, acne is very distressing.

Diet is important and sweets and oily foods must be avoided. It is important to stay away from junk food, takeaways and dairy products; nuts and chocolate can also cause problems. Drink soy milk as a milk substitute and get plenty of fresh air and exercise to help keep the skin healthy. Foods containing high levels of vitamin A have shown good results with acne sufferers as have foods with high zinc content. As teenagers' diets are usually not as good as they should be, supplementation of these nutrients is advised.

Skin care needs special attention. It is best to avoid removing blackheads as this may result in scarring. It can be done if the area has been softened with a special lotion containing the herb thyme. Only soaps designed for skin health should be used and a good skin scrub will help remove the dead top layer of skin and help open the pores. This will allow the sebum to escape without clogging. To treat the pimples use a tea tree gel daily. Tea tree is an anti-bacterial oil which will not harm healthy skin but will effectively destroy acne bacteria. Also, wash and condition the hair regularly and keep it off the skin as this will aggravate the oiliness.

TOPICAL TREATMENT
Wash face with an anti-bacterial face wash daily.
Apply a tea tree gel to the pimples once daily.

SUPPLEMENTS

	children over 12
Bio Zinc	1 tablet daily with food
cod liver oil	1 teaspoon daily before food
vitamin E	250iu daily with food
sodium sulphate	200mg twice daily

In severe cases add echinacea 175 mg twice daily in combination with red clover, sarsaparilla, burdock and yellow dock.

Ageing and slowing down the visible signs

Have you ever wondered why some people look so young? When we are born our time clock starts ticking the years away. Genetic factors set the base but we cannot choose our parents.

There is a hypothesis that our time clock is housed in the mitochondria, or the powerhouse of each cell. One theory is that when the mitochondria are damaged by the attack of toxic free radicals over a period of years, eventually they are unable to withstand this onslaught and they die, causing the death of the cells. It is therefore important to reduce or exclude foods from the diet that contain high levels of free radicals. These free radicals are a by-product of oxygen metabolism, or form as the result of eating certain foods. Oxidised fats are considered one of the highest sources of free radicals and many believe that these rancid fats could indeed be one of the major causes of cancer and heart disease. It is the antioxidants in our bodies that control the excess free radicals, preventing them from damaging and destroying healthy cells, thus decreasing the visible signs of ageing.

Cardiovascular disease, which includes heart attacks and strokes, is the number one killer of Australians. Hardening of the arteries is a contributing factor in cardiovascular diseases which can result in high blood pressure, angina and certain types of senile dementia. The good news is that, through dietary changes and supplementation with antioxidants, it may be possible to slow down the progress of arteriosclerosis (hardening of the arteries) and help prevent some of these killer diseases.

Evidence has shown that the taking of antioxidants may indeed extend the quality and length of life and reduce the incidence of many other diseases. Dietary antioxidants consist of a number of nutrients including vitamins C, E and beta-carotene, the mineral zinc and the amino acid methionine.

Have you ever noticed that a cigarette smoker usually has a more heavily lined face (especially around the mouth) than someone who doesn't smoke? Smoking causes free radicals to form. These can damage the skin and they also reduce the level of vitamin C in the blood. The nicotine in cigarettes constricts the blood vessels leading to the surface of the skin, robbing it of nutrients and therefore causing the skin to become malnourished and dry. This can indeed lead to the early signs of ageing.

Stopping smoking is an obvious solution but what about side-stream smoke, pollution and photochemical smog? If you are exposed to these pollutants then you will require more antioxidants in your diet. An easy way of ensuring that your dietary antioxidants are at a level that is sufficient to reduce free radical damage is to take a supplement. I would suggest that a quality vitamin A, C and E antioxidant formula be part of your everyday support regimen.

Hormonal imbalances and faulty enzyme metabolism may also be a cause of premature ageing. These hormonal changes, in particular the changes that occur as a woman approaches menopause, are the causes of thickening and coarsening of the skin. The addition to the diet of evening primrose oil which contains essential omega-6 fatty acids can help correct these problems. These fatty acids have a direct effect on the prostaglandin pathway, indirectly balancing hormones and improving the texture and softness of the skin. I would suggest supplementing the diet with one 500mg capsule three times daily.

Water is a must. Consume between 6 to 8 glasses of water each day either by drinking water or eating foods containing water, such as whole fruits. This helps flush your body of toxins and keeps your skin supple.

Every day it is important to exercise. Exercise improves the blood flow to the muscles and organs, increasing their tone and reducing sagging. For the best results exercise for 20 minutes daily, bringing your heart rate up to 75 per cent of the maximum heart rate for age. This can be determined by taking your age from 180. An example would be if you are 50 years old then your maximum heart rate to achieve is 130 beats per minute. It is best to see your practitioner before undergoing any exercise program just in case there is an underlying disease of which you are not aware.

Although a suntan may make you look brown and healthy, it dries and damages your skin, prematurely ageing it. You should keep out of the sun as much as possible and definitely avoid sunbaking and sunburn. Whatever the colour of your skin, do not allow your skin to burn, and apply moisturisers to it every day.

Moisturisers, fats and oils have been applied to skins by all cultures since the beginning of time in an endeavour to improve the skin's texture and appearance. The external treatment of your skin is just as important as supplementation.

As we age, without proper care, the skin's cells become thicker, larger in appearance and harder. The dead layers of skin that we shed rapidly in youth are now much more difficult to shed.

The use of an exfoliating scrub will remove the layers of dead skin and speed up the process of regeneration. This should be followed by daily skin care treatment including toning, moisturising and nourishing.

Finally to help slow down the ageing process think young. Yes, your mental attitude is an important factor. If you think old, then old you will be.

SUPPLEMENTS
an antioxidant formula containing beta carotene, vitamin C and vitamin E

evening primrose oil	500mg 3 times daily
zinc	12mg daily
selenium	50 - 100 mcg or as prescribed by medical practitioner

Allergies

An allergy is the body's reaction to a certain substance that is foreign. The substance that triggers an allergic reaction in a sensitive person is called 'an allergen'. This could be found in pollen, dust, hair, fur, an insect bite or sting, certain foods, medications, plants, and other sources. Food allergies in children are common. Babies and children may be allergic to cow's milk or dairy products (see also ALLERGY TO COW'S MILK, Part 1). If this is the case then try substituting goat's milk or soy milk. Conditions including asthma and eczema are often the result of an allergic response to allergens in the air or to foods and/or chemicals (see also ASTHMA). Avoid foods containing sulphite, amine and salicylate which can cause allergies and may need to be restricted in the diet. If this is the case then remove these foods group by group.

Establish the level of the food group by avoiding eating any of the foods listed under any one of the food groups known as salicylate, amine or sulphite for a period of 5 weeks. You may now add these foods to the diet but this must only be done one food at a time. If the food causes any problems or a recurrence of symptoms then discontinue this food for three months before trying again.

Foods containing sulphite

The following food additives are mainly found in the list of foods mentioned below: sulphur dioxide (220), sodium sulphite (221), sodium bisulphite (222), sodium metabisulphite (223) and potassium metabisulphite (224).

frozen avocado
pickles and pickled onions
sausages and sausage mince
red wine, cider and (in small amounts) beer
potato crisps and hot chips
dried vegetables and instant potato
some cordials, soft drinks and dessert toppings
uncooked prawns

Migraine headaches may be the result of eating hard cheese, chocolate or oranges. This type of headache can be reduced by up to 90 per cent by observing diet restrictions.

Your practitioner can carry out the following tests to determine allergies. The cytotoxic blood test compares the reaction to as many as 120 different types of foods. The results will help you determine the foods that might need to be eliminated from your diet.

Also the RAST (Radio-Allergo Sorbent Test) can be very useful in determining allergies to animal dander, dust mites, moulds, fungi and grasses.

Foods that are high in salicylates

HIGH	VERY HIGH
sweets	
	liquorice
	peppermints

HIGH	VERY HIGH
	honey
herbs and spices	
cinnamon	cayenne
cardamon	aniseed
black pepper	sage
ginger	mace
allspice	paprika
clove	thyme
	mint
	Vegemite
	mustard
	Worcestershire sauce
alcohol/beverages	
coffee	Nature's Cuppa
	Coca Cola
	decaffeinated tea
	liqueur
	port
	fruit juice
	wine
	rum
fruit	
	passion fruit
	sultana/date
	mulberry
	prune/date
	grape
	raisin (dried)
	currant (dried)
peach	cherry
watermelon	apricot
	Jonathon apples
	orange/rockmelon
	Granny Smith apples
	strawberry
	pineapple

HIGH	VERY HIGH
vegetable	
eggplant	tomato
watercress	tomato products
cucumber	gherkin
broadbean	endive
alfalfa	champignon
capsicum	radish
avocado	olive
nut	almond

Foods that are high in amine

sweets	milk, white and dark chocolate
condiment	
bonox/Vegemite	Marmite
	meat extracts
beverages	beer, port, wine, sherry
meats, chicken and fish	
bacon	beef, liver, pork
	fish marinades
	sardines/tuna
cheese	most cheese
vegetables	sauerkraut, spinach
nuts	
macadamia	walnut
	black walnut
	pecan

SUPPLEMENTS
children 12 years and over

vitamin C and the	1,000mg morning and night

bioflavonoids	lowers elevated blood histamine levels
vitamin E (natural)	500iu daily with food has anti-histamine properties
vitamin B6	25mg daily with food may help reduce sensitivity to MSG
children 6 to 12 years	take 1/2 (50%) of above

Alzheimer's Disease

Alzheimer's disease accounts for around 50 per cent of all senile dementia sufferers and without doubt, as we grow older, this form of dementia is the most dreadful. This disease is distinguished by a steady and progressive loss of memory due to the deterioration of brain function, and wasting. This deterioration is also associated with the presence of tangles of fibres and plaques within the brain nerve cells.

Alzheimer's disease may begin at any age after forty but is most likely to affect individuals over fifty years of age. Over the years a better understanding of this disease has been gained, but with all our modern technology and knowledge, modern medicine still has no answer to its treatment and/or cause.

There are many theories regarding the cause of Alzheimer's disease, ranging from genetic deficiencies to slow acting viruses and although these may have merit, I believe that nutritional deficiencies and toxic mineral accumulation over the years could be the key to the cause of Alzheimer's disease and other types of senile dementia.

Eating correctly from a variety of foods each day is a must because the diet is the main source of essential nutrients, including vitamins and minerals, needed to maintain a healthy body and mind. Many studies have shown that patients suffering from dementia are deficient in one or more of the important vitamins or minerals and if their levels are too low the result can be dementia.

Dietary supplementation with antioxidants including beta-carotene (pro-vitamin A), vitamins C and E and the minerals zinc and selenium could be vital in protecting the brain from free radical damage, a possible cause of dementia and premature ageing.

Vitamin E has been shown to be deficient in nearly 60 per cent of Alzheimer's sufferers. This essential vitamin is a powerful antioxidant. Vitamin E also helps to maintain a healthy vascular system and reduces the viscosity (thickness) of the blood, reducing the incidence of blood clots in the brain, a major cause of CVA (stroke).

A reduction in blood flow and oxygen to the brain can be caused by the narrowing and hardening of the arteries leading to, or in the brain, and this is a major cause of senile dementia. Prevention of this process is imperative if a normal state of memory and mind power is to be preserved as the years go by. Supplementing the diet with an antioxidant formula containing natural beta-carotene, vitamins C, E and K, along with the mineral zinc, will ensure that these important nutrients are included in your daily diet.

The herbs *Ginkgo biloba* and ginseng have been shown to be of benefit in the treatment and prevention of senile dementia. Clinical studies have found that the ancient herb *Ginkgo biloba* (maiden hair tree) has a positive effect on the mental performance and vigilance of the elderly. This herb also helps to improve the memory by increasing the blood flow to the brain and its uptake of carbohydrates. *Ginkgo biloba* is available from health food stores and pharmacies and could be valuable in the treatment and prevention of many types of dementia including Alzheimer's disease.

The ancient Chinese valued the herb ginseng more than gold. It was said to slow down the ageing process, improve the memory, the concentration and the zest for life. Ginsana, a concentrated herbal extract of ginseng, has undergone many clinical trials, the results of which indicate that the Chinese were correct in their evaluation of this ancient and valuable herb.

Garlic has been used as a medicinal and culinary herb since ancient times and is a valuable cardiovascular tonic. Studies have shown again that history was correct in the use of this herb over the centuries. The action of fresh or freeze-dried garlic can be beneficial in many ways. Investigations into garlic show that when it is taken on a regular basis it can help to lower cholesterol and blood pressure which can be responsible for strokes and diseases such as hardening and narrowing of the arteries, one cause of dementia.

Garlic should be included in the daily diet, but if the smell is a problem look for a garlic supplement that has an enteric coating that allows the garlic to be ingested in the intestine and not the stomach ... result: all the advantages of the whole garlic herb without the smell.

High aluminium levels have been detected in the brain cells of patients who suffer Alzheimer's disease, so many researchers believe that aluminium could be a factor in the cause of the disease. Some of these studies question the use of aluminium based antacids and deodorants as these can cause elevated aluminium levels within the body.

The herb slippery elm is very effective in relieving the symptoms of gastric reflux, heartburn and ulcer pain; symptoms that many people would seek to relieve by using aluminium based antacids. There are also alternatives to aluminium based anti-perspirants which are available from health food stores; choose one of these instead.

Five steps to improve your memory

1. Eat a well-balanced diet, high in fibre and low in animal fats.
2. Supplement with an antioxidant formula daily.
3. Include ginkgo, garlic and ginseng in the daily diet.
4. Avoid the use of all aluminium products.
5. Keep active both mentally and physically; the mind needs exercise too. Remember it's never too early to start; prevention is always better than cure.

Anaemia

Anaemia is a condition in which the number of red blood cells in the body is reduced. The symptoms of anaemia range from tiredness, paleness of the skin and in particular the fingernail beds, and a feeling of weakness, to just not feeling 'quite right'. There are three main classifications of anaemia: when the bone marrow, where red blood cells are made, does not produce enough of these red blood cells; when the body destroys an excessive number of red blood cells; when the body suffers a loss of blood, as may occur from heavy menstrual cycles, bleeding haemorrhoids or from other undetected internal bleeding.

Anaemia may also be caused by vitamin deficiencies and a lack of iron in the diet. Vitamin B12 and folic acid are essential for the production of red blood cells and without either a condition called macrocytic anaemia will occur in which the blood cells become larger than usual. Pernicious anaemia can cause a deficiency in vitamin B12. This in turn can affect the brain and the nervous system.

During pregnancy vitamin B12, iron and folic acid are essential for the mother's health and the child's development. Supplementation may help prevent anaemia in pregnancy and also neural tube defects in the developing fetus. Good food sources of these nutrients are liver, kidney, yeast, deep green leafy vegetables, asparagus, broccoli, lentils, lima beans, whole grains, mushrooms, egg yolk, lean beef and veal.

Supplementation for mother and child is necessary as folic acid can be destroyed in cooking and canning processes. Vitamin C is also important as it markedly enhances non-heme iron absorption and is beneficial when taken for the prevention and treatment of iron-deficient anaemia. Other clinical studies have also found that supplementation with other B group vitamins could be of advantage in the treatment of many types of anaemia.

SUPPLEMENTS

15mg iron phosphate	take 1 with food 3 times daily
vitamin B12	4mcg daily with food

multi vitamin and mineral (sustained release)	1 tablet with food each morning
folic acid	0.5mg daily or as prescribed
vitamin C	1000mg with food twice daily

Anal fissures

This complaint will upset your children and make them very unhappy. The discomfort is equal in pain to an adult case of haemorrhoids. Fissures are a tear at the opening of the bowel. These tears may bleed slightly and are very painful, especially when your child passes a motion. Fissures are usually caused by constipation. The passage of the constipated, dry, hard stool causes tearing of the anus. Anal fissures can also be caused by the child scratching the area, usually because of irritation caused by worms. Diarrhoea can be another cause.

Treatment involves cleaning the area after going to the toilet and having a bath in warm salty water three times a day. The salt is antiseptic and reduces the swelling. If constipation is the cause then increase the fibre in the diet. Include fresh vegetables, fruit and whole grains. Water is also important so encourage the sufferer to drink more.

TOPICAL TREATMENT

A lotion made up as follows will heal the fissures quickly if used 3 times daily.

wool fat	6 parts
liquid extract of witch hazel	1 part
soft paraffin	3 parts

SUPPLEMENTS

| psyllium husks | 2 teaspoons mixed in with cereal or juice |
| vitamin C and bioflavonoids | 1,000mg added to the daily diet |

Anorexia nervosa **and bulimia**

Anorexia nervosa usually develops in young women and is thought to affect around 2 per cent of the population.

The symptoms are a loathing of body fat and a fear of weight increase. This can lead to extreme dieting and in some cases, self-induced vomiting (bulimia).

The causes are varied but family problems and peer pressures have an effect. Girls who are pressured to achieve academically, or who strive to be slim and beautiful, are at risk. Anorexics get a distorted view of their own bodies, seeing themselves as fat even when thin.

It is important at this time to show love and understanding. However, never treat the problem lightly. If you suspect the problem contact your medical practitioner.

Bulimia nervosa is a disease occurring mainly in young women and has similar symptoms to *Anorexia nervosa* but differs in that the sufferer, in some cases, does not look undernourished. Bulimics tend to gorge themselves and then induce vomiting. In this way they keep their weight stable.

The risk bulimics run is ulceration of the oesophagus, damage to the teeth caused by the stomach acids and a lack of vitamins and minerals.

Studies have shown that a lack of zinc in the diet could be a contributing factor in anorexia and bulimia. Also clinical evaluation of anorexics found a deficiency of essential fatty acids.

If the disease is diagnosed, counselling is advised. A supportive group called Overeaters Anonymous can be found in the telephone book.

SUPPLEMENTS
children over 12 years of age

zinc	25mg per day with food
multi-vitamin mineral	1tablet with food daily
evening primrose and fish oil combined	2 capsules with food twice daily

spirulina   as a food additive
alfalfa   380mg dried herb 3 times daily

Arthritis

Arthritis (see also FISH OIL) has a number of causes and can start at any age. It is an inflammation of the joints accompanied by pain and swelling. There are many forms of arthritis. However rheumatoid arthritis, gout, and osteoarthritis are the main forms.

Osteoarthritis affects the hips, knees, and shoulders and is part of the ageing process but it can also affect other joints such as in the spine and hands. Gout is a form of this where uric acid crystals form in the joints. These two forms of arthritis are rare in children and adolescents.

Rheumatoid arthritis, also known as Still's Disease, is a disease of the connective tissue and commonly occurs in the young. It is thought to be a disease of the auto-immune system in which the body produces a disordered immunological response. The symptoms include swollen joints, skin rashes, enlarged lymph glands, and possibly enlarged liver and spleen.

Children may run a temperature of 40°C for several weeks and develop an inflammation of the tissues around the heart and lungs. They will become lethargic and complain about not feeling well. They may even develop abnormally, commonly developing a receding chin line.

Children between the ages of 2 and 12 can develop arthritis and it is more common in girls than boys. It is a debilitating and chronic disease with long term treatment which is aimed at relieving the symptoms and stopping the joints deteriorating.

To alleviate the pain and reduce the discomfort, diet is very important. A diet low in fats and moderate in the intake of protein is the first step. Avoid all organ meats such as liver, kidney, brains, heart, and sweetbreads. Do not eat shellfish of any kind, preserved meats such as salami, tinned fish, oranges and tomatoes. Plenty of milk, eggs, fruit and vegetables, butter and wholegrain or stoneground breads (avoiding whole wheat) should be the basis of the child's diet.

Do not give aspirin. Reduce red meat consumption to three times a week but eat steamed chicken or fish as often as desired. Supplement this diet with a B complex, vitamin C, pantothenic acid and a cod liver oil supplement. To keep the body flushed of toxins, drink 6 to 8 glasses of water per day.

Fish oil has been shown to help in the relief of the pain of arthritis as it has anti-inflammatory properties. The herbs celery seed and guaiacum are very useful as they also have anti-inflammatory properties.

Recent scientific studies have found celery seed extremely helpful. Celery complex relieves the inflammation and helps detoxify the joints. White willow bark acts as an analgesic as it has similar properties to aspirin without many of the side effects.

Exercise is a great benefit to pain relief and encourages healing but should be restricted to non-jarring activities such as swimming and walking.

SUPPLEMENTS

Celery Complex	children 6 - 12 years one tablet with food morning and night 12 years to adults, 2 tablets with food 3 times daily
celery extract	follow directions on bottle
fish oil 1000	children 6 - 12 years one capsule mixed with food twice daily over 12 years and adults up to 4 capsules daily with food
multi vitamin and mineral	1 daily or as directed

To help reduce pain and fever use a formula containing:

white willow bark	2700 mg children 6 to 12 years

up to 3 daily
adults and children over 12
years up to 6 daily

Asthma

The word asthma (see also FISH OIL) comes from the Greek for 'panting'. It is a chronic inflammatory disease that is accompanied by wheezing and shortness of breath. During an asthma attack the mucous membranes swell and the bronchial tubes go into spasm, breathing is an effort and the exhalation of air from the lungs becomes more and more difficult. In children this is a very frightening and even terrifying experience.

There are two main types of asthma. One is 'intrinsic asthma', which usually develops in conjunction with an infection, or later in life, and may follow the birth of a child or change of life. Extrinsic asthma is the other and is caused by allergies.

In young children who suffer with asthma the cause is usually an allergic reaction to certain foods. Cow's milk, artificial colours, artificial flavours and preservatives are some of the known causes of asthma in babies and young children. These foods, or food additives, should be excluded from the diet. Fresh is best and fresh foods should be your first choice. If this is not always possible (as may be the case with feeding babies) then canned foods would be the next choice as they are preserved by heat. Always read the label of the can carefully and look for a product that does not contain any additives. Substitute soy bean milk for cow's milk, as soy bean protein is more easily digested and does not usually cause any allergic reactions.

There are other foods that may cause an adverse reaction and clinical studies have shown that egg, fish, shellfish and nuts (in particular peanuts) can cause the immediate onset of asthma. Delayed onset of asthma may be caused by chocolate, wheat, citrus fruit and colourings, in particular tartrazine (yellow dye food additive number 102).

Other foods such as those high in amine or salicylate (see also ALLERGIES) could also be the cause of allergic symptoms such as asthma. Unfortunately many individuals may suffer from multiple allergies, and if this is the case then time will be needed to establish all allergy problems. Asthma attacks may also be caused by small particles of feathers, pollen, dust, mould, animal dander, air pollution and fly sprays. These allergens can aggravate the bronchial tubes in sensitive children or adults, causing an asthma attack.

The medical management of asthma is with the use of bronchodilators and anti-inflammatory drugs. The main bronchodilating drug used is Salbutamol (Ventolin) and this drug is administered with the use of an inhaler (puffer) or in a nebuliser.

Salbutamol relaxes the muscles that surround the bronchial tubes causing them to dilate and make breathing easier. This type of medication is very helpful and used by most asthmatics. Side effects of Salbutamol can be anxiety, fine tremor in the hands and restlessness.

Another drug commonly used in the medical treatment of asthma is Beclomethasone (Becotide). This drug is a corticosteroid and has a direct marked anti-inflammatory effect on the inflamed bronchial mucosa. Beclomethasone is prescribed usually when the use of bronchodilators is inadequate in the control of asthma. Possible adverse effects of Beclomethasone include irritation to the throat and nose caused by fungal infection. This can be managed by gargling with warm water with a little salt and one drop of tea tree oil added. The prolonged use of corticosteroids at high doses may also affect the normal functioning of the adrenal glands. If adverse effects occur then these should be discussed with your medical practitioner.

Possible link between asthma deaths and medically prescribed drugs

Possible over-treatment as reported in the *Australian Doctor* (p.23, 6 February 1987)

Some possible reasons put forward were the excessive use of bronchodilator aerosols, particularly the potent 'Isoprenaline Forte' used in many countries.

One other suggestion put forward as a possible cause of the more recent increases in death rates, especially in New Zealand, was a possible cardio-toxicity effect of combinations of beta-adrenergic agonists and methyl xanthenes, especially in older people.

Letter in the *Lancet* (p.161, 17 January 1987)
The increased mortality from asthma seen in the UK and in the USA has coincided with the introduction of new means of overcoming attacks — namely, aerosols with selective beta-adrenergic effects.

Letter in *New Scientist* (27 July 1991)
The strongest warning so far of the dangers of some asthma drugs, including the widely used brands Ventolin and Berotec, has been sent to regulatory bodies world wide. In a confidential letter, Boehringer Ingelheim, the German company that makes Berotec, warns that people who inhale these beta-2 agonists face an increased risk of dying from asthma.

Naturopathic management
The naturopathic management of asthma is not to discontinue prescribed medication but to remain free of symptoms with the use of supplements, diet and herbs, therefore reducing the requirement for stronger medication.

Diet
A vegetarian diet excluding all meat, dairy products, fish and eggs showed significant improvement in 92 per cent of asthma sufferers. This diet also excluded chlorinated tap water, sugar, coffee, salt, apples and citrus fruits; these fruits are high in salicylates (see also ALLERGIES).

As vegan diets are usually low in iron and vitamin B12, supplementation of the diet could be needed. In this case it would be wise to talk to your naturopath or medical practitioner.

Supplementation with vitamin C can help. Vitamin C appears to have an anti-asthmatic effect. Vitamin C can also help reduce the symptoms of the common cold and improve resistance to infection.

| children | 500mg daily for children 6 to 12 years of age |
| adults | 1000mg vitamin C combined with the bioflavonoids morning and night |

One of the most useful herbs is liquorice. This herb has a corticosteroid action similar to that of beclomethasone. The active constituents of liquorice include glycyrrhizin, with steroid-like effect which gives it its anti-inflammatory action. Liquorice has long been used in herbal medicine for the treatment of many bronchial complaints. Large doses over a long period of time may cause sodium retention and potassium excretion. Potassium intake should be increased and a low sodium diet followed.

| children 6 to 12 years | 500mg of liquorice twice daily before meals |
| adults | 1,000mg just before meals 3 times daily |

The inclusion of the simple onion or garlic in the diet will help improve resistance to colds and flu. These two foods should not be overlooked as they are really good for you. Studies have also found that these good foods may help reduce the asthmatic response to airborne allergens. Eat fresh garlic and onions daily. If the taste or smell on the breath is too strong then take a garlic supplement.

| odourless garlic | 6 to 12 years of age 50mg equivalent to fresh garlic with food morning and night |
| freeze-dried garlic | adults 1 tablet equivalent to 2,000mg fresh garlic before food each night |

The herbs euphorbia and grindelia have been used traditionally in the treatment of asthma. Grindelia has antispasmodic effects that help relax the bronchioles, relieving mild asthma attacks. Euphorbia is mentioned in the *British Herbal Pharmacopoeia* as an anti-asthmatic herb and when used for the treatment of asthma is best taken with grindelia. A tablet containing 220mg of euphorbia and 220 mg of grindelia is recommended twice daily for children 6 to 12 years, 3 times daily for adults, with food.

The addition of cod liver oil to the diet may also help. Cod liver oil contains vitamin A. This vitamin helps strengthen the mucous membranes in the lungs. Also cod liver oil contains essential fatty acids that have an anti-inflammatory effect. Cod liver oil has been used for generations in the treatment of many bronchial conditions.

children 6 to 12	2.5 mls (1/2 teaspoon daily) just before food
adults	5.0mls (1 teaspoon) daily just before food

If the asthma attack is accompanied by acute bronchitis then drinking three or four cups of thyme (*Thymus vulgaris*) tea daily will not only help relieve the asthma attack but also soothe the bronchioles.

children 6 to 12	half adult dose
adults	1 cup of the infusion made from the flowering apical bud 3 to 4 times daily

It must be noted that many asthmatics have multiple allergies and even the foods, medicine or herbs that help prevent asthma may also cause problems. For this reason it is best to begin any changes slowly, adding new medications or dietary changes one by one and noting the reaction. Never stop taking your practitioner's or naturopath's medication without consulting them first.

Athlete's Foot

Athlete's foot is a fungal infection that can affect children from any age. However it is more common in children from school age onwards than it is in babies. The fungus is everywhere in our environment and can quickly take hold if proper care is not taken. The most important precaution is to keep the feet dry and clean. The fungus that can cause athlete's foot needs a moist area to live and the ideal place is between the toes.

The fungus is contagious and is found in gyms, swimming pool change rooms and locker rooms. It is best to advise your children to wear thongs when entering these areas.

TOPICAL TREATMENT

The treatment for athlete's foot is firstly to kill the fungal infection. This can be done by washing the area in a diluted tea tree oil solution - a commercially available wash is one used for acne, Antibacterial Face Wash, by Blackmores. Wash the feet in this wash morning and night then dry the area using a hair dryer on low heat. Don't let young children use hairdryers unattended.

The area should then be powdered with a cornflour and zinc oxide powder which will keep the feet dry and prevent the reinfection of the area. Some people seem to be more vulnerable to fungal infection than others. I have found that supplementing the diet with vitamin C, zinc and acidophilus and bifidus improves resistance to this infection. The diet should be a high roughage, complex carbohydrate diet, low in dairy products, low in yeast, with virtually no refined carbohydrates.

SUPPLEMENTS

Vitamin C	children 6 to 12 take 250mg or chew half a tablet with food morning and night adults 1000mg with food morning and night
children's chewable multi vitamin	chew 1 tablet with food every morning
bio zinc	25mg of zinc with food every morning
acidophilus and bifidus	take one capsule just before main meal each day

Bad breath or halitosis

The cause of bad breath has to be found before it can be treated. Causes range from poor oral hygiene, constipation, to sinusitis and bronchitis. When either mucous or pus builds up in the airways, it creates a foul smell. The most common causes of bad breath are poor oral hygiene and digestion.

If the source is the mouth then it is most likely to be the teeth. Proper brushing and flossing of the teeth will remove rotting food matter that becomes lodged. This rotting food not only can cause bad breath but also tooth decay.

Children are often unaware of the necessity for correct brushing technique and need to be trained and supervised, using dental floss and brushing. Plaque which builds up on the teeth houses bacteria that can also cause bad breath and increase tooth decay.

Herbs can help. If the problem is caused by the digestive system, the breath becomes worse when the stomach is empty. Supplement the diet with acidophilus and bifidus or eat acidophilus yoghurt which will help the growth of healthy friendly bacteria and balance gut flora.

A little chlorophyll or peppermint tea will also help freshen the breath and improve digestion. It is very important to drink plenty of fresh water daily. This will also aid digestion, help flush toxins from the body and promote good health (see also CONSTIPATION). Charcoal tablets can help, as can Digestive Bitters if indigestion is the cause.

Bad breath may be the result of other problems including infected tonsils, adenoids, sinus congestion or bronchitis.

SUPPLEMENTS

acidophilus and bifidus	1 tablet just before meals each night
chlorophyll	as directed on the bottle

Bedwetting

Bedwetting is a problem that affects up to 10 per cent of

children over the age of five. True bedwetting is when the child consistently wets the bed after the age of five. It is quite normal for a child to wet the bed during illness or if overtired. Don't make a fuss about this problem, or try to shame the child into not wetting the bed at night.

Most children grow out of this habit quickly but if it continues there may be an underlying physical disease causing the problem. Urinary tract infections, diabetes, abnormality of the urinary tract or a nervous condition may be the cause of children's bedwetting.

To treat the condition first try rewarding your child for good behaviour and never become annoyed or angry as this will only cause problems with the relationship between you and your child. Have a talk to your practitioner about persistent bedwetting. Your child can be examined to determine if the bedwetting is caused by illness. If no illness is detected, and the problem continues, then without making a fuss encourage your child not to drink large amounts of fluid between dinner and going to bed.

The diet should include fresh fruits and vegetables which will help maintain a healthy urinary tract and prevent the urine from becoming acid. Encourage your child to drink water upon arising and throughout the day, only restricting water intake after dinner at night. With a well-balanced diet supplementation with a children's multi vitamin may also be of benefit.

Sodium phosphate, a natural cell salt, is known as the fluid mineral. In conjunction with potassium chloride it helps maintain the acid/alkaline factor in the blood. Also sodium sulphate helps regulate kidney function and these two celloid minerals can help prevent bedwetting.

Professor Rudolf Weiss, a German medical doctor and herbalist, found that St John's wort is useful in the treatment of bedwetting and night terrors in children. Corn silk also helps control bedwetting. It may be labelled on the health food store shelf under the botanical name *Zea mays*.

SUPPLEMENTS
sodium phosphate   4 to 8 years 1 crushed

	tablet containing 200mg of sodium phosphate at night
childcare chewable multi vitamin	4 to 10 years 1 tablet daily with morning meal
St John's wort	add 1 teaspoon to 1 cup of water, boil briefly
	4 to 6 years of age, drink 1/4 of a cup morning and night
	6 to 10 years of age, drink 1/2 of a cup morning and night
corn silk complex	4 to 8 years 1 tablet containing 800mg of *Zea mays* twice daily

Birthmarks

About 50 per cent of infants have birthmarks or skin blemishes at birth. These usually disappear during the first or second years of life. These marks may be salmon-coloured, red, blue-black or purple in colour; other forms of birthmarks are strawberry marks, portwine marks and pigmented moles.

Strawberry birthmarks may develop during the first 4 to 5 weeks and affect 10 per cent of infants. These marks are a result of small blood vessels packing closely together. They are most often raised and may stand out when the child cries. This type of birthmark usually fades completely by the time the child is 6 years. Pigmented moles and portwine birthmarks usually do not fade and may be permanent.

There is no treatment needed for birthmarks. However, strawberry marks may become infected if the skin is broken. If you notice any unusual odour or discharge from a birthmark it is best to discuss this with your practitioner.

Tea tree oil or a cream containing comfrey extract, natural vitamin E and apricot kernel oil will usually heal the area quickly. The bioflavonoids and vitamin C will help strengthen the capillaries and improve the tone of the blood vessels. This may help prevent any minor ruptures.

SUPPLEMENTS
vitamin C
multi vitamin and mineral formula

Bites and Stings

Life in Australia exposes us all to insect bites and stings, the effect of which depends on the biter and the person. If the person has a history of allergic reaction then urgently seek medical aid.

Bee stings are usually left behind in the skin with the venom sac. The first thing to do is remove the sting by scraping it sideways with your fingernail or a blunt knife. Clean the area and then apply cold compresses.

Mosquito bites are best prevented with the use of a fan, citronella or tea tree oil, or a mosquito net. If bitten, then treat the itch with bicarbonate of soda or tea tree oil.

Sandfly bites are extremely irritating and can be prevented by taking a vitamin B group supplement.

European wasp may sting several times but does not leave the sting behind. The symptoms of the sting are extreme pain and swelling of the air passage. Wash the area clean and apply cold compresses. If there is any sign of an allergic reaction then urgently seek a medical practitioner, check the pulse and breathing and apply mouth-to-mouth resuscitation if necessary.

Bluebottle stings in summer are a hazard. If stung, remove the tentacles with tweezers or the fingers and apply cold compresses. If a large area of the body is affected, then seek medical advice.

Box jellyfish are found in tropical waters between October and May and protective clothing is advised as well as the carrying of 4 litres of vinegar. Do not dive into the water and if stung retreat slowly. Pour vinegar on the stung area for 30 seconds and if possible apply ice. Resuscitation may be necessary and breathing and consciousness must be checked continually. Get medical aid immediately.

Funnel web spider is found on the New South Wales and southern Queensland coasts, is reddish brown to black, 2 to 3 cms in length and lives in burrows, holes, crevices, trees and underneath houses. If bitten, place a pressure immobilising bandage beginning at the bite and covering the whole limb. Rest and reassure the casualty. Seek medical attention immediately.

Red back spider is found throughout Australia and is identifiable by the red stripe on the back. It lives in old tyres, buckets, pots, and garden sheds, and these habitats should be cleaned regularly. If the spider bites, reassure the casualty, apply a cold pack and urgently seek medical aid. Do not bandage area.

Snakes are very shy and only attack when provoked. Be noisy when walking in the bush and wear stout shoes and socks. If bitten, leave the venom on the skin for identification and do not cut the bitten area. Use a pressure immobilisation bandage beginning at the bite and covering the whole limb. Rest the patient and seek medical aid urgently.

Ticks occur throughout Australia and can be venomous and cause paralysis, or not be as venomous and only cause skin irritation. Remove the tick by sliding small scissors or tweezers on each side of the tick and levering it out. Be careful not to leave the mouth in. Check the body crevices for other ticks and if the casualty is a child, or if the sufferer is nauseous and sick after a tick is found and this feeling lasts, then seek medical attention.

Blisters
Blisters can be painful and may become infected, particu-

larly if they break. A blister is a reaction of the uppermost layers of the skin to injury from pressure or heat, or to a virus or bacteria.

Burns can cause extensive blistering and should be treated by a medical practitioner if the area burnt is on the face, hands or genitals. Any severe burn or a burn or blistering that covers a large area of skin needs professional treatment. Do not break the blister. It will break naturally as the skin underneath heals. Prevention of infection is vital. Small pressure blisters on the feet need to be treated with an antiseptic such as tea tree oil, golden seal or calendula and covered with a sterile non-stick dressing. For blisters on newborn babies see NAPPY RASH and for blisters on the mouth see COLD SORES.

If blisters are caused by a burn place the area under running water as soon as possible. Following this treatment apply aloe vera gel either straight from the plant or in a formula to the area. It will heal both the burn and the blister very quickly.

Blood poisoning

Blood poisoning (septicaemia) is serious in children and should be treated urgently by a medical practitioner or hospital as it can be fatal. Blood poisoning is caused by certain bacteria entering the bloodstream, or by their toxic by-products (see also TOXAEMIA Part I). This may be the result of skin penetration by a nail or dirty object, through to an abscess on the lung or burst appendix. The affected person's symptoms may include fever and chills, delirium, irritability or lethargy.

As the poisoning advances, the blood pressure may decrease, breathing slows down, the pulse becomes weaker, skin may be covered by a bluish coloured rash and become clammy to the touch. Unconsciousness and coma can occur. If blood poisoning is not quickly treated, damage to the heart, brain, bones and liver, can occur.

SUPPLEMENTS
Must be managed by a practitioner. However, supplementing the diet with extra vitamin C, 1 teaspoon of cod liver oil daily

and the herb echinacea will help strengthen the immune system and may indeed help prevent septicaemia.

Bloody nose (see Nosebleed)

Boils

Children often get boils and these can be particularly painful. Most boils are a staphylococcal infection of the hair follicle or sebaceous gland. The most common places for boils to form are on the face, the back of the neck, lower back or under the arms.

It is very important not to pick at, squeeze or pierce the boil as this may spread the infection causing further boils. If the infection enters the bloodstream it can be quite serious. Use a hot compress and poultice to draw the boil to a head and to relieve pain.

To make the poultice, use equal parts of slippery elm bark powder, marshmallow and burdock leaves. This should be applied to the boil and changed regularly during the day. Any pus should be cleaned up and disposed of properly and the area cleaned with antiseptic before re-dressing.

When the immune system is compromised, infections including boils can and do develop. It is therefore very important to ensure that your child's diet is well balanced and should include at least 3 pieces of fruit per day, a variety of cereals, fresh leafy green vegetables, orange vegetables, fish and eggs. Avoid too much fat in the diet. Supplementing the diet with extra vitamin C and the herb echinacea will help increase immunity to infection and boils.

Celloid minerals such as silica help remove waste from the body and potassium chloride and iron phosphate reduce inflammation and fight infection.

SUPPLEMENTS

vitamin C	children 6 to 12 years
	250-500mg daily

echinacea complex
175mg dried herb
or liquid extract

children over 12 years
1,000mg daily
children 6 to 12 years 1
tablet with food morning
and night
children over 12 years
1 tablet with food 3 times daily
For extract follow directions on
bottle.

Bowels (see Constipation and Diarrhoea)

Breast cancer

Breast cancer frightens many women. It must be realised that breast cancer can be treated but remember prevention is better than cure. There are many dietary factors that have been linked to the disease. A diet high in vegetables containing beta-carotene has been shown to be related to a low incidence of breast cancer. Diets low in fat decrease the incidence of breast cancer. Make sure your diet is well balanced.

Around 70 per cent of your diet should come from complex carbohydrate — fruit, vegetables and whole grains, about 10 per cent to 13 per cent from protein, and the remainder from fat. Unfortunately many Australians eat as much as 50 per cent fat in their diet, increasing the chance of breast cancer.

Vitamin C is important in the diet and can block the formation of nitrosamines in the intestines and stomach. These nitrosamines are carcinogenic and are formed in the body from everyday foods. Amines, combined with nitrates and nitrites, form these deadly substances (see also IMMUNE SYSTEM). Vitamin C can protect the body against these nitrosamines and other carcinogens.

Fish oil has been found to suppress cancer in women in high risk groups. Dr George Blackburn, Associate Professor of Surgery at Harvard Medical School, says he would be dumbfounded if fish oil did not thwart the spread of malignant cells in women who undergo breast cancer surgery. He believes the fish oil may strengthen immunity, killing wandering cancer cells before they start new tumours.

Environment is also important. Avoid cigarette smoke even if you are not a smoker. Side-stream smoke from another person's cigarette can cause cancer.

It is important to regularly examine the breast and make sure no lumps or physical differences to your usual body shape have appeared. If there are changes, do not delay seeing your medical practitioner. There is a lot that can be done. Naturopathy is preventative. If you have cancer you will need medical management in conjunction with supplements and balanced diet. Delay can reduce the success of the treatment.

Pretending it is not there will not make it go away. A positive attitude to health is beneficial.

SUPPLEMENTS

fish oil	1,000mg 3 times daily
antioxidant formula containing	
vitamin A, C, E and zinc	1 daily
selenium	50-100mcg daily or as directed by medical practitioner
garlic	2,000mg fresh herb equivalent each night
beta-carotene	6mg daily

11 STEP ANTI-CANCER PLAN

1. Do not smoke.
2. Balance low fat and high fibre in diet.
3. Eat only organically grown fruit and vegetables.
4. Maintain weight for height.
5. Reduce or quit alcohol consumption.
6. Stay out of the burning sun.
7. Supplement diet with essential fatty acids and antioxidants.
8. Reduce all stressful experiences.
9. Avoid carcinogens such as benzine, nicotine

and saccharin.
10. Be positive about yourself and your life.
11. Carry out regular breast examinations.

Breast Self-Examination

(adapted from the NSW State Cancer Council)
Every woman should become familiar with her breast structure so if a change does occur it will be noticed. A woman's risk of developing cancer is 1 in 15. Cancers under 2cm in diameter, when detected and treated, may have little effect on life expectancy. The surgery, if detection is early, is unlikely to be a mastectomy (removal of the breast). If you do find a lump, do not panic. The chance of it being cancer is 1 in 10.

If you are over 25, examine your breasts once a month on the first day after your period. If it is after menopause, then do it on the first day of each month. Run your fingers clockwise and anticlockwise around the breast getting to know its peculiarities. Each breast is different. If you feel a thickening, lump or abnormality, go and see your medical practitioner.

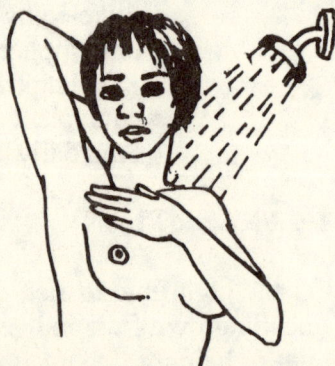

In the shower, soap the breast, lift the elbow and put the hand behind the head. Using the flat of your hand and in a gentle and relaxed manner, examine your breast in quarterly segments. Alternatively, examine the breast in widening circles from the nipple outwards. Examine right up to the armpit.

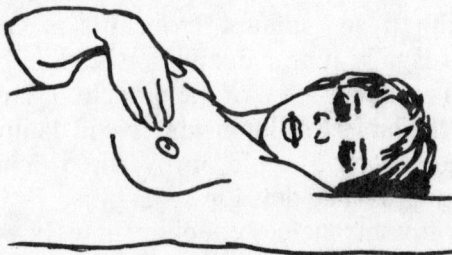

If lying down suits you because of softer or larger breasts, place a pillow under your right shoulder and put your right hand behind your head. Follow the above for the process of examination. Be aware not to mistake your ribs for lumps.

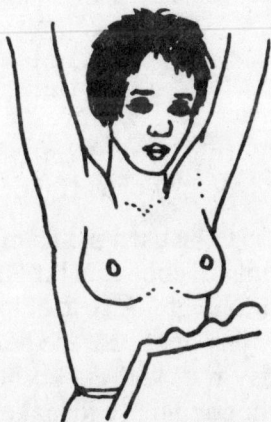

Looking in the mirror you may notice something you missed in physical examination. Look for differences in the contour of the breasts and irregularities such as puckering or retraction of the nipple. Use 3 different positions —arms by side, arms raised above the head, with arms pressed hard on the hips to tense the hip muscles. If your breasts are large, lean forward to get a better look at the contours.

Bronchitis

In children and infants, bronchitis is very often acute whereas it is usually a chronic condition in adolescents and adults. Bronchitis is inflammation of the bronchi or large air passages that lead to the lungs. Children who live in damp environments, eat poorly, are exposed to cold, are overtired, or who have caught a cold or flu virus may develop bronchitis.

The symptoms include coughing at night which is initially unproductive but may develop and produce thick yellow phlegm, noisy rattling coughing, and a fever. At night, when the coughing is at its worst, use a vaporiser (either a commercial brand or a bowl of boiling water which can hold its heat). To these add vaporiser liquid. You can make your own vaporiser liquid (see below) or there are many brands to choose from in health food outlets.

Vaporiser liquid - each 5ml contains:

camphor	250mg
eucalyptus oil	0.5ml
wintergreen oil	0.1ml
menthol	500mg
tea tree oil	0.2ml

in a base of propylene glycol to 100 per cent

The above liquid is to be used in steam vaporiser units for the treatment of the coughs of colds and bronchitis. This will ease breathing and loosen the phlegm. Also to help loosen phlegm and soothe the inflamed air passages, use the herbs liquorice, horehound, mullein, pleurisy root and euphorbia. In combination, these will help relieve the coughing and make it more productive.

Cod liver oil has been used for decades for colds, flu and bronchitis. The essential fatty acids in the oil have an anti-inflammatory effect and the vitamin A helps strengthen the mucous membranes. Garlic, vitamin C, and echinacea will help prevent further infection.

SUPPLEMENTS
vitamin C   2 to 6 years 100mg daily

	6 to 12 years 250mg daily
	over 12 years 1,000mg daily
cod liver oil	children 2 to 6 years 1.5mls
	6 to 12 years 2.5mls daily
	over 12 years 5mls daily

a liquorice complex containing liquorice, marshmallow, slippery elm, senega and grindelia

> children 2 to 6 years 1/2 tablet morning and night in food children 6 to 12 years 1 tablet morning and night, over 12 1 tablet with food 3 times daily

Bruises

We can all bruise and it is caused by the rupturing of tiny blood vessels under the skin after a blow or bump. The pain of a bruise can be relieved by using cold compresses of fresh water and ice. Do not use salt water as it will further damage the bruise. If a child goes to bed without bruises and wakes up with them, or bruising occurs without reason, then discuss this with your practitioner.

The best way to treat a bruise after applying cold packs is to use the herb arnica. A tincture of ointment made from the herb is used for external application to sprains, bruises and wounds. Children who bruise easily should be encouraged to eat more fruit and vegetables. Supplementing the diet with bioflavonoids and vitamin C can strengthen the blood vessels and help prevent bruising.

SUPPLEMENTS

vitamin C	over 12 years 1,000mg tablet once daily
Chewable	6 to 12 years 2 tablets daily
Vitamin C	under 6 years 1 tablet in food daily

Bulimia (see *Anorexia nervosa*)

Burns

Unfortunately children burn themselves accidentally. There are many causes of burns including sun, chemicals, fire, electricity, friction, boiling water and steam.

Serious burns should always be treated by a medical practitioner and are often coupled with shock and infection. If the burn size is larger than a 20 cent piece, or involves the face, hands or genitals, it is serious.

There are two main classifications of burns - the first are deep thickness burns which affect the deeper tissue. The area burnt may look white or black and charred. Often there is no pain as the nerves that sense pain have been damaged or destroyed. Superficial burns are on the surface, are red and may have blisters. For all burns, run cold water on the burn for 10 to 30 minutes, depending on the severity. Do not apply oily lotions of any kind, do not give any alcohol, only small sips of water, do not break any blisters and do not put on dressings which will stick to the burn. If the burn is serious a medical practitioner's help should be sought immediately.

As the burnt skin recovers, or if it is not serious, it needs to be treated to aid healing and promote recovery. The best known herb for this is aloe vera which can be taken directly from the plant and applied to the skin. A commercial gel is available which helps cell regrowth. Zinc is a mineral which aids healthy skin and is an important supplement. Vitamin C is important also for the health of the skin's collagen or 'cement'. Vitamin E helps prevent scarring.

SUPPLEMENTS

zinc	6 to 12 years 6mg daily
	12 years and over 12-25mg daily
vitamin C	6 -12 years 250mg daily
	12 years and over 1 tablet daily
vitamin E	12 years and over 100iu daily

TOPICAL TREATMENT

| aloe vera | apply to the burnt area after treating with cold water |
| vitamin E cream | apply alternately with aloe vera to help prevent scarring |

Candidiasis (Candida or Thrush)

This infection is also called candida, monilia or thrush and is caused by a yeast-like fungus called *Candida albicans*. It can occur in the vagina, the mouth, the intestines and on the skin. It is caused by changes in the body's chemistry which destroy the body's immunity and encourage the fungus to grow. Taking antibiotics can create the right environment for the fungus to grow, as can diarrhoea. In females it most commonly occurs in the vagina and anus, causing itchiness and a white discharge. In males it occurs around the anus, and in babies it occurs around the nappy area and in the mouth (see also NAPPY RASH).

For thrush in the mouth use a little diluted tea tree oil on a cotton bud. Wipe on the affected area and then wipe again with a clean cotton bud to remove excess residue. It is necessary to have a diet low in sugar and refined carbohydrates, dairy products and foods containing yeast. A *Lactobacillus acidophilus* supplement will help your child recolonise gut flora which has been unbalanced by the fungus.

The inflamed area can be soothed with diluted tea tree oil which has powerful anti-fungal properties. Zinc oxide and cornflour powder should also be applied after the area is completely dry.

More information about candida and its treatment for adults can be found in *Get Well An A-Z of Natural Medicine for Everyday Illness*.

SUPPLEMENTS

| acidophilus and bifidus | babies and children take a supplement with meals or goat's milk yoghurt twice daily |

| enteric coated | over 12 years and adults take |
| garlic | 1 tablet before food each night |

Cardiovascular disease
(see Immune system)

Chickenpox

Chickenpox is a viral infection that mainly affects children. However, adults can still contract the disease. Babies up to six months old are immune from the disease but it is best not to allow contact with children who have chickenpox when it is in the contagious stage.

What to look for if you suspect chickenpox: your child may feel unwell or seem to have a slight cold the day before any rash appears. This starts as a red spotty rash and is itchy. The rash soon becomes raised and forms pimples which become blisters. In about 4 days the blisters form scabs. This process continues until the whole rash has formed crusts.

As chickenpox is a highly contagious disease, your child should be kept home from school and away from other children until the rash has formed scabs and any fever has gone. The disease can be transferred to other children by droplets from the nose or mouth when they talk, cough, sneeze, or by direct contact with the rash or sores. The first symptoms of chickenpox usually appear between 12 to 21 days after contact with an infected person.

Secondary infections can occur if your child is allowed to scratch the sores. Keep the fingernails short and the hands and nails clean at all times. This will minimise the risk of secondary infection occurring. To help stop the itching use the following mixture combined with water. Apply this paste to the itch.

STOP ITCH FORMULA

zinc oxide	1 part
bicarbonate of soda	1 part
cornflour	1 part

It is best to keep your child in bed until the temperature has subsided. Give the child plenty of fluids and keep the diet light. To help keep the temperature down lightly sponge your child with a cool cloth on the forehead and back of the neck.

Do not give the child aspirin as it has been associated with Reye's Syndrome, an illness which can be life threatening. In very rare cases inflammation of the brain (encephalitis) can be a complication of chickenpox. If there is high fever, vomiting or convulsions see your medical practitioner.

Echinacea, red clover, sarsaparilla are all useful herbs to give your child. They have a blood purifying action helping rid the body of infection. Echinacea also stimulates the immune system and is mentioned in the *British Herbal Pharmacopoeia* as an anti-viral herb.

Vitamin C helps the body fight infection and build the immune system. Vitamin C is not stored or manufactured in our bodies and must be consumed in our diet daily. Fresh fruits and vegetables are a good source of vitamin C.

SUPPLEMENTS

echinacea tablet or liquid extract	2 to 6 years 1 tablet containing 175mg crushed in food daily 6 to 12 years 1 tablet containing 175mg with food morning and night
vitamin C	2 to 6 years 75mg morning and night with food
chewable vitamin C	6 to 12 years 250mg tablet morning and night

Choking

A mother's nightmare is to discover her baby, or infant choking on a bottle top, peanut or other unwelcome object. A foreign object in the upper airway is an immediate threat to life.

If the object is visible, probe with your finger to remove it by placing the infant on your forearm. If the child is able to speak and is conscious, ask the child to cough. This may force the object out. Try to get the child to relax and breathe deeply. If the child is unable to breathe or is unconscious, turn the head face down on your knees and give four blows between the shoulder blades to propel the object out of the windpipe. If this fails, maintain the airway and carry out expired air resuscitation. Quickly seek medical assistance.

Cigarette smoking

Cigarette smoking has been promoted by advertisers as a desirable image of sophistication, elegance, success and maturity. It has unfortunately captured the imaginations of many teenagers who think smoking is grown up. Once hooked, people depend on cigarettes for stimulation, stress relief, weight control, or it becomes an uncontrollable habit. Unfortunately men appear to be smoking less while women appear to be smoking more, and they start during adolescence.

As people reject the image of smoking and give up, the burning issue of passive smoking arises. Non-smokers become subjected to side-stream smoke which is the smoke which comes directly off the cigarette and seems to have a magic ability to go straight up the non-smoker's nose. According to research, the side-stream smoke has more toxins than smoke drawn through the filter, making passive smoking a real health threat and doubling the dangers of smoking.

If your child or you smoke then you increase the risk of cancer by 25 times, depending on the length of time you have smoked, and the risk of cancer of the throat and mouth by 10 times. You double the risk of heart disease (and the risk is even higher if you are a woman taking oral contraceptives), and you will almost certainly contract chronic bronchitis and increase your chances of catching colds, flu and sore throat. You shorten your life by 5 minutes with each cigarette you smoke. Pregnant women run a higher risk of miscarriage and giving birth to a stillborn baby and their baby will be smaller and perhaps less intelligent. Disorders of the circulation and coldness of the extremities can lead to degeneration of tissue.

Giving up? The best way to start is with a juice fast. This method helps the body cleanse itself by increasing the capacity of the lungs, liver, kidneys and skin to eliminate toxins. This elimination of poisons and metabolic waste from the body also helps remove the desire to smoke.

As large amounts of vitamin C are destroyed with smoking, it is advised you supplement your diet while smoking and after giving up. Research done by Dr Gary Duthie of Rowett Research Institute of Aberdeen, Scotland, indicated that smokers are under higher oxidant stress than non-smokers and this stress can be partially compensated for with vitamin E supplements.

If calming the nerves is your smoking excuse, try a formula containing the herbs passiflora, scullcap, valerian and hops in combination with a B group vitamin formula. This will calm your nerves and decrease the desire to smoke. Your children, hopefully over 18 years, will also benefit from these herbs. After giving up smoking you then need to repair the lungs. Take cod liver oil which contains vitamins A (essential for healthy mucous membranes) and essential fatty acids in combination with vitamins E and C.

SUPPLEMENTS

antioxidant formula	over 15 years 1
with vitamins A, C, E	tablet morning and night
formula of passion-flower, hops, valerian, scullcap	
Smoke Stop	homeopathic formula that removes desire to smoke, place drops under tongue

Cold sores *(Herpes simplex)*

The herpes virus is related to chickenpox (see also CHICK-ENPOX) and is highly contagious. As with chickenpox, it first appears as painful nodules, then blisters, then pustules, followed by scabs. The *Herpes simplex* virus comes in two forms. Type 1 usually appears as cold sores around the mouth. Type 2 is genital herpes which occurs on male and female genitalia and which is sexually transmitted. Both types are contagious in the period when the sores or lesions are apparent, just forming or just healing. This may cover a 2 week period and great care should be taken to avoid passing the virus on as it is difficult to cure and recurs.

Pregnant women may pass on the infection to the unborn child in the placenta, but more commonly during childbirth by way of the infected vagina. Infected babies have a high risk of congenital abnormalities of the central nervous system and the brain. It is difficult to treat as drugs may be more life-threatening than the disease.

As treatment is difficult, the most effective way to manage the illness is to attend to diet and lifestyle. Vitamin B foods such as fresh, leafy, green vegetables, whole grains, liver, yoghurt, sunflower seeds and a good quality B complex are important.

The dietary aspect of treating herpes is centred on two amino acids: arginine and lysine. Under laboratory conditions the virus grows well if supplied with arginine whereas lysine inhibits growth. Avoid foods highest in arginine - chocolate, nuts, carob, buckwheat, whole wheat and cooked oatmeal. Eat foods high in lysine such as fish, shellfish, chicken, beef, cheese, all kinds of beans, milk and eggs. Stick to this diet and take a lysine supplement. Zinc is also proving of great importance in treating this disease. Echinacea is a herb which stimulates the immune system and has anti-viral properties.

Rest, relaxation and sleep are very important to control stress. Stress will bring on an attack very quickly and stress management is critical. A Canberra psychologist, Magdulski (1981), used relaxation therapy and self-hypnosis on 39 patients with herpes and followed them up for 14-37 months. None of the 39 had a recurrence. Exercise and fresh air also contribute to peace of mind and good health.

SUPPLEMENTS

l-lysine	children over 12 and adults 500mg

	twice daily
vitamin C	1 tablet twice daily (containing 1,000mg of vitamin C)
zinc	1 tablet daily with food (containing 12mg of elemental zinc)
echinacea	500mg of the dried herb 3 times daily
acidophilus and bifidus	take 1 tablet before meals twice daily

Lypsine contains a mixture of the above in one formula.

Colds and flu

Most children at one time or another will catch a common cold. Colds are caused by many different types of viruses and it is these viruses that infect the nose, throat and upper respiratory tract causing pain, congestion and fever.

Commonsense tells us that keeping warm and avoiding behaviour which involves sudden temperature changes, such as leaving a warm house to play in the cold outdoors, will help prevent the common cold. These sudden changes in temperature lower resistance to infection in children. Correct nutrition is also a necessity. Recent studies and clinical trials have shown that vitamin C (found in fruit and vegetables) can help strengthen the immune system, reducing the incidence and symptoms of colds and flu.

Children need to eat fresh fruit and vegetables daily, as vitamin C cannot be stored nor can it be manufactured by our bodies. Scientific evidence also suggests that supplementing a well balanced diet with extra vitamin C could further improve the body's resistance to infection.

Vitamin C supplementation can start with bottle fed babies. Blackcurrant juice is one of the best sources of vitamin C. Rose hip formulas which are also high in vitamin C are readily available. These fruit juice formulas should be included in babies' daily feeding routine. Children over 2 years can either have a crushed Chewable Vitamin C tablet added to their food or chew one tablet twice daily. Herbal medicine is also helpful when used to treat and prevent infections. The herb echinacea has anti-viral properties and stimulates the immune system. When combined with garlic it destroys the invading viruses.

Cod liver oil is another nutrient that has been used for decades in the treatment of cold and flu. This fish liver oil contains fatty acids that help reduce inflammation and make breathing easier. Also cod liver oil is a good source of vitamin A. This vitamin is needed to help strengthen the mucous membranes (see also EARACHE for information on nasal sprays and BRONCHITIS for vaporiser liquid formula). A vaporiser is of great help at night when you and your child are sleeping. Don't forget grandmother's remedy of a few drops of eucalyptus on the pillow at night and on a handkerchief in the day to clear the nose and make breathing easier.

SUPPLEMENTS

vitamin C	children 6 months to 12 months vitamin C baby formula as directed
	1 to 6 years 100mg
	6 to 12 years 250mg daily
	12 years and over 1000mg
cod liver oil	6 months to 6 years 2.5 ml mixed in milk
	6 years and over 4ml daily
Echinacea Complex	6 - 12 years 1 tablet daily
	12 years and over 2 tablets
Children's Herbal Cough Syrup	1 to 12 years 2.5-5ml 3 to 4 times daily
Honey and Herbal Cough Mixture	over 12, 5ml every 4 hours
Cold Tablet formula with iron phosphate and and potassium chloride	follow directions on bottle

Colic

Despite the fact that simple colic usually disappears of its own accord as the child grows up, it can cause parents and baby much distress at the time. Rapid feeding, gulping air, fermenting food in the stomach, stress, allergy or poor digestion can all cause colic.

When colic occurs, lay baby across your knees on its stomach and gently rub its back. Sometimes a hot water bottle filled with warm water, placed on the distended tummy can help. Colic attacks can also be relieved by helping stimulate bowel movements. Use a glycerin suppository to pass gas from the bowel. If it is diagnosed as a milk allergy, switch to a soy bean or goat's milk. The same applies to the mother if she is still breastfeeding the baby.

The best old-fashioned method is gripe water or dill water tea. To make your own gripe water take 1 teaspoon of dried dill seeds and 1 teaspoon of dried peppermint. Add 1 cup of boiling water and a pinch of sodium bicarbonate. Cool and filter.

newborn babies	2.5 to 5mls
6 months to 1 year	10 to 20mls
1 year and over	20 to 30mls

Concussion

A bang on the head caused by a car accident, diving into shallow water, playing football or just falling over - all can lead to the state of being concussed. Concussion is a state of altered consciousness, or unconsciousness, following a blow to the head. When a child is unconscious, lay the child on its side, ensure he or she can breathe, be alert to the possibility of an injured spine, put no pressure on any part of the skull, and if bleeding from the ear is occurring, lightly place a sterile dressing on the ear and lay the injured child side down. Always refer to medical aid if the child has lost consciousness, even for a short time. When the child goes to sleep it is wise to check by waking the child every 2 hours to make sure that all limbs are 'working' and all other functions are normal. If the child starts to convulse or the pupils are uneven (not the same size) or they are vomiting, behaving in an unusual manner or are difficult to arouse, seek medical attention urgently.

Conjunctivitis

Many irritations can cause the upsetting condition called conjunctivitis. The conjunctiva covers the eyeball and lines the eyelid and can become inflamed as a result of a virus, bacteria, a foreign body, allergy or even long exposure to artificial lighting, as is the case with those who work indoors under fluorescent lights. Bacteria may only affect one eye whereas a virus will usually affect both eyes.

A herbal tonic to treat this condition is a combination of golden seal and eyebright. The herb bayberry can also be included in this formula. To make the eyewash, add 800mg of the dried golden seal herb to 1 cup of boiling distilled water. Let it stand for 20 minutes then filter through a paper coffee filter and bathe the eyes twice daily.

Supplement with the herb echinacea as it stimulates the peripheral blood vessels and the immune system and helps the healing process.

Constipation

Constipation in children is common. The first rule in managing constipation in your child is to have an understanding of the problem. Many parents confuse constipation with regularity, indeed the two are all too often thought of as one, but this is not the case. Constipation is directly associated with the hardness of the stool (motion) and not the frequency. Although a stool movement daily, or more, is desirable for the elimination of toxins from the body, a normal healthy child may have less than one movement per day if the metabolism is slow. If the stools are soft and normal, then constipation is not the problem even if the child is only passing one motion every second day.

Constipation in children is usually a result of either poor

diet or the child resisting the call to nature. If your child is constipated then the diet needs to be closely looked at. Increase the amount of fibre in the child's diet; whole grains, fruit and vegetables are all good sources. Apples and bananas are best restricted if the child has constipation as these fruits can worsen the problem.

A resistance of the call to nature results in constipation because the bowel absorbs the water from the retained stool, resulting in the stool becoming hard and difficult to pass. If this is the problem, it is important not to scold the child if he or she soils their pants during toilet training. Scolding will only worsen the problem; the child will associate normal bowel movements with being unclean and will resist the call, resulting in further constipation.

Water helps lubricate the stool and is therefore very important. Many children unfortunately do not drink enough water. Encourage the child to increase the intake of water. By the age of 12 your child should be drinking 6 to 8 glasses of water per day. Herbs also can help. Cascara, senna and cape aloes in combination (these can be found in the herbal formula Peritone) stimulate bowel movement. It is best not to rely on laxatives to treat constipation. Instead, try to improve the diet and increase fluid intake.

If the child is constipated for some time then a condition known as paradoxical diarrhoea may develop. This condition is associated with watery stools and a hard round stool in combination in a single motion. This may seem to make the diagnosis of diarrhoea difficult, however this type of motion should be considered constipation.

SUPPLEMENTS

water	6 to 8 glasses per day
psyllium husks	over 4 years, 1 teaspoon in juice morning and night
magnesium complex	1 tablet with food twice daily
Peritone formula	6 to 12 years 1 tablet every second night

Croup

Croup is a barking cough which can readily alarm parents when it affects their babies and young children. It occurs as an acute inflammation of the upper respiratory tract but may also occur as a complication of laryngitis, diphtheria or whooping cough.

It usually is not serious but can be frightening and this may cause the spasm to worsen. The way to assess the severity of the croup is to listen to breathing when the coughing has stopped. If it is still noisy then talk to your practitioner.

The best way to immediately soothe the problem is to humidify the air. A vaporiser is excellent. There are many types available. It is the inhalant that is important. Make it up yourself or use a formula containing menthol, eucalyptus, wintergreen oil and camphor (see also BRONCHITIS).

SUPPLEMENTS

euphorbia herb	children 1 to 6 years take 1 tablet crushed in food at night children 6 to 12 years of age take one 220mg tablet with food twice daily
children's chewable vitamin C	children 1 to 6 years 1 daily children 6 to 12 years 250-500mg daily with food

Crying

Crying is baby's way of telling you something is wrong. They may be hungry or frightened, suffering colic, just plain irritable, or wanting attention from parents. Teething is also a common cause of crying. Crying is your baby's or child's way of getting attention. It is infant power and the child's only way of communicating. Do not try and stop the child crying; it is a release. Try and find the reason and offer comfort to the baby or child. Often this will solve the problem (see also COLIC, CONSTIPATION, NAPPY RASH)

Cuts and abrasions

Everyone collects a variety of cuts and abrasions which need immediate care to avoid infection and scarring. Light cuts can be treated with a wash in an antiseptic solution and clean or sterile non-stick dressing. If a deep cut occurs, control the bleeding by applying pressure to the wound. If bleeding is under control, clean the wound as well as possible. If you have a sterile dressing, apply it to the wound and seek your practitioner's help. Wash your hands, do not cough or sneeze on the wound and avoid handling it except with clean or sterile dressings. Only remove foreign objects if they have not penetrated the tissue and can be brushed or washed off. Whether or not you attend a doctor, remember that a person with a penetrating cut may need a tetanus injection.

If a penetrating object such as a large nail or fish hook is embedded in the flesh, pad around it and then bandage the padding into place, rest the limb and quickly seek medical aid. Do not attempt to remove it yourself, do not apply any pressure to the object and do not try to shorten it unless its size is unmanageable.

Abrasions go hand in hand with skateboarding and riding a bicycle. Dirt may become embedded in the wound and cause infection. Clean the wound with a sterile dressing soaked in cool boiled water and use an antiseptic to help prevent infection. Dress the abrasion with a non-stick bandage.

TOPICAL TREATMENT
tea tree oil, golden seal, echinacea and calendula in ointment form can all prevent infection
Vitamin E healing cream will help prevent scarring
Keep the wound clean and dressed until healed to prevent infection.

Cystitis

Cystitis is an inflammation of the bladder and can be caused by bacteria entering the body through the urinary tract. This may occur in several ways. This condition is more common in girls than in boys, as girls have a shorter urethra or urinary tract allowing the infection to enter the area more easily. This infection is not as common in young children as after puberty and into adult life.

Symptoms of the disease can include a frequent need to urinate even with little or no result, and burning and painful urination. The urine may have a strong, fishy smell, and as it may contain pus, is usually cloudy in appearance. Real cystitis can occur when a woman does not completely empty her bladder, leaving a residue of urine which may become infected and cause cystitis. During pregnancy most women find they need to urinate more frequently. This need is caused by the developing fetus placing pressure on the bladder and, this in turn, can cause retention of urine with the resulting problems.

If you or your child is suffering from cystitis and it is accompanied by a fever or is not responding to treatment, then see your practitioner.

To treat cystitis, always wear cotton underwear and keep the genital area clean and dry. Drink 6 to 8 glasses of water a day to keep the kidneys and bladder flushed, eat alkaline foods, restrict red meat, eggs and whole wheat. Also spicy and hot foods should be avoided as they can irritate the bladder. Herbal teas which will soothe the urinary tract include corn silk, boldo, marshmallow, couch grass and bearberry. Also drinking barley water, an old remedy, can be of great help.

SUPPLEMENTS

herbal complex containing cornsilk 400mg with bearberry, buchu and couch grass	as directed on bottle
celery 300mg and juniper 200mg	children over 12 years 1 tablet with food 3 times daily adults 1 to 2 tablets 3 times daily

Dermatitis and eczema

Broadly speaking, dermatitis and eczema are both skin disorders which can be similar in appearance and are usually caused by allergies. The two types of skin disorders are external.

Dermatitis can be the result of a reaction to an external irritant such as household detergent, nylon, chemicals or an infection. Dermatitis on the hands is common and as it may be related to an external allergen, it is known as 'occupational' or 'housewives' dermatitis'.

Eczema is usually associated with, or related to, an allergy and is the more common of the two in children. Children who suffer from eczema often suffer from other allergic conditions such as asthma. The symptoms of eczema may manifest themselves from the age of 6 months, often first appearing as a rash on the cheeks or small weeping cracks behind the ears. This condition can worsen and become generalised eczema in which the whole body may become affected by the rash which can become crusty, weeping and very itchy. The medical management of these conditions may include antihistamines and compounds which give symptomatic relief but do not solve the problem.

Treatment naturopathically involves the patient avoiding the allergens that quite often are causing the condition. Also controlling or avoiding stressful situations can help as these can precipitate an outbreak. Ointments containing chickweed, pine coal tar, and juniper berry can help reduce inflammation and stop itching and help reduce inflammation. One such ointment is Eczema Balm, another is Chickweed Compound.

Diet also plays an important part. Foods rich in vitamin A and zinc are helpful as are the herbs sarsaparilla, red clover, burdock and dandelion. These herbs have been used traditionally in the treatment of many skin conditions. Evening primrose oil is of help in many skin disorders. One double-blind crossover study reported in the *Lancet* pp. 1120-22, 20 November 1982, showed that supplementation with evening primrose oil reduced overall severity of eczema by 43 per cent. Clinical studies have also shown that cow's milk and eggs aggravate the condition in a number of children.

SUPPLEMENTS

Efamol evening primrose oil	children 1 to 2gms daily adults and children over 12, 1 to 3gms daily
vitamin A	follow directions on bottle
zinc	children 6 to 12 years 6 mg tablet daily over 12 years one 22mg tablet daily

TOPICAL TREATMENT

Chickweed Compound	apply twice daily
Eczema Balm	apply when needed

ZINC CREAM

anhydrous wool fat	3ozs
olive oil	3ozs
zinc oxide	4ozs
solution of lime	4fl ozs

Apply to the affected parts as required.

ZINC CREAM

For young children and infants

zinc oxide	6gms
corn starch powder	6gms
crude coal tar	1gm

Mix with soft paraffin to make 1 ounce.

Diabetes

Diabetes is a disease in which people cannot metabolise carbohydrates because the pancreas will not secrete insulin, the hormone which regulates the metabolism of blood sugar. It is thought that the disease is hereditary. Half a per cent of children suffer from diabetes mellitus and the onset is usually sudden and severe. The child or adolescent loses weight, gets hungry and thirsty constantly, urinates frequently and has a dry and itchy skin. Treatment is essential as the final outcome could be diabetic coma.

The 2 types of diabetes mellitus are insulin independent and insulin dependent. It is the latter which tends to occur in adolescents and it is sometimes called juvenile onset diabetes. Sufferers depend on insulin injections and must be under the care of a medical practitioner.

Research has shown that vitamin and mineral supplementation can help sufferers. Chromium is a component of the glucose tolerance factor (GTF) and it increases tolerance in animals, boosting the effectiveness of insulin. It is found in brewer's yeast. A high fibre, high complex carbohydrate diet including foods such as cereal grains, especially rolled oats, root vegetables and legumes is important. Avoid any refined sugars. Complex carbohydrates should be 75 per cent of the diet, protein 15 to 20 per cent, and fat 5 to 10 per cent. Clinical studies have found that zinc is excreted in the urine by diabetics. A zinc supplement may be useful.

Clinical studies have also shown that vitamin C improved glucose tolerance in patients given 500mg daily. Supplementation may be useful but if your child is supplementing with vitamin C it may alter the results of urine tests. Talk this over with your medical practitioner who must also be supervising the disease.

SUPPLEMENTS

Brewer's yeast	for children over 12 years
	500mg twice daily
vitamin C	1,000mg daily
zinc	25mg daily
vitamin E	100iu daily

Diarrhoea

Diarrhoea in children is characterised by watery and loose

motions, not the frequency of the bowel movements. Diarrhoea can occur from a variety of causes. Some of the most common are infections of the digestive tract including gardia, amoebic and bacillary dysentery, coliform and staphylococci; or reactions to food or medication. Some of the foods that may cause diarrhoea in children are cow's milk, prunes, corn products and oranges.

Cow's milk unfortunately can be a problem for many children, as an allergy to the protein may develop at an early age. If this is the case soy or goat's milk may solve the problem. Lactose (sugar of milk) intolerance is another cause of diarrhoea. This is caused by a lack of the enzyme lactase in the intestine, resulting in an inability to absorb the lactose, and leading to diarrhoea. Lactose intolerance can be genetic or it may follow a gastro-intestinal infection. The signs and symptoms to look for if diarrhoea is suspected may include loose and watery stools, cramps and fever. There may also be spots of blood and mucous.

Diarrhoea in babies and very young children can be dangerous and must not be left unattended as dehydration may result. A loss of 5 per cent or more of a baby's weight due to diarrhoea could be an indication of serious dehydration. Hospital treatment of this condition may be necessary.

If the condition is caused by an infection then both the diarrhoea and the infection need to be managed. Extra fluids to drink and mineral waters with added glucose are best. Restrict all fruits, vegetables, whole grain and high fibre foods. Apples and bananas can be given and don't seem to cause any problem. Give the child dry foods to eat when starting back on the normal diet.

If infection is still present then further treatment may be needed. Also the intestinal flora will need balancing. The addition of garlic followed by acidophilus can help restore normal bowel bacteria. It should be noted, however, that garlic can upset some individuals and should not be given in large amounts to young children.

The herb echinacea can also be helpful in combating infection; even young children can take this herb. Speak to your naturopath about the dose for your child or follow the directions on the bottle.

SUPPLEMENTS

Agrimony Complex	6 to12 years one 300mg tablet morning and night
slippery elm	6 months to 2 years 300mg in food morning and night 1 to 6 years 300mg twice daily 6 to 12 years 1 to 2 tablets before meals 3 times daily

Dizziness

Dizziness is also called vertigo and it is a feeling of spinning or moving sideways. It can be accompanied by nausea, vomiting and cold sweats. The problem could be quite serious, coming from the balancing mechanisms in the brain or the middle ear. Tinnitus, or ringing in the ears, may set in. If this is the case then see your practitioner. In adolescents it is more likely that dizziness would be a result of an inner ear infection (see also EARACHE), or low dietary iron intake, especially with teenage girls. Inner ear infections can be picked up by swimming in polluted water. Another cause is motion or travel sickness (see also MOTION SICKNESS).

SUPPLEMENTS

If as a result of low dietary iron:

iron compound	12years and over, one 15mg tablet with food 3 times daily

If as a result of inner ear infection:

echinacea	175mg dried herb 3 times daily
vitamin C	1,000mg daily
cod liver oil	2.5 to 5ml daily before food
horseradish and garlic	1 tablet just after food 3 times daily

Dyslexia

Between 5 per cent and 10 per cent of children are thought to be affected by dyslexia which is a difficulty in recognising written language. Boys are 4 times more prone to the disorder than girls - one school of thought is that boys have only one side of the brain with a language centre whereas girls have them on both sides of the brain. Frequently confused letters are 'b' and 'd', and 'q' and 'p'. Some children have difficulty writing, playing games, and telling their left from their right. Conversely they may be very good at maths, reading music and memorising poetry.

New research carried out at the University of Miami School of Medicine in Florida for the National Institute of Child Health and Human Development in Washington found that there were fundamental differences, in particular a size difference between the rear portion of the left hemisphere of the brain in normal readers which is larger, compared to that of dyslexics. Magnetic resonance imaging also revealed that the corpus callosum, a band of nerve fibres connecting the two hemispheres of the brain, was much larger in dyslexics.

The problem for parents is to detect it if it is present as it may affect the way the child performs at school. Dyslexia will not affect intelligence or eyesight but it may affect performance if the child feels inadequate without knowing why. Remedial teaching helps enormously.

The herb ginkgo improves blood circulation to the brain and short term memory, and the celloid minerals potassium phosphate and magnesium phosphate, help improve nerve transmission and concentration.

SUPPLEMENTS

Ginkgo biloba	12 years and over 500mg dried herb twice daily
potassium phospate and magnesium phosphate mineral formula	1 tablet 3 times daily

multi vitamin and mineral
sustained release formula   1 tablet daily with food

Earache (Ear infections)

By the time children have reached the age of 6 years, up to 95 per cent will have suffered an ear infection. Objects of small size inserted in the ear may become lodged in the ear canal or the eardrum may be injured if a sharp item is pushed into the ear. The two most common causes of ear infections are otitis externa (outer ear infection) and otitis media (middle ear infection), the more common of the two.

Severe earache occurs with this infection that usually starts with a blockage of, or infection in, the eustachian tube. This infection can be passed along from the throat. Occasionally tooth decay can be the source of earache as can a boil, or sinusitis. One of the first signs of earache in young children is pulling at their ear in an attempt to relieve the pain. They also usually develop a fever and become nauseous.

Initial treatment involves placing a warm hot water bottle wrapped in cloth under the ear, while the patient is lying down. Three drops of warm garlic oil placed in the child's ear will help relieve the pain and infection. Fever should be reduced by sponging with cool water. The herb white willow bark works like aspirin in reducing fever and relieving pain.

If the problem is recurring, supplement the diet with cod liver oil, echinacea, garlic and vitamin C to build the immune system and fight infection. If the condition does not improve then antibiotics may need to be prescribed by a medical practitioner.

SUPPLEMENTS

Echinacea liquid extract	all ages as directed on bottle
cod liver oil	1 to 6 years 2.5 ml daily with food or in milk
	6 to 12 years 4 ml daily
vitamin C	1 to 6 years 100mg daily with food

6 to 12 years 250mg daily
with food
12 years and over 1,000mg
 tablet twice daily

NASAL SPRAY FORMULA
To make a child's nasal spray take 1 teaspoon of salt and 1 teaspoon of glycerine and add to 600ml of boiled water. This can be placed in an empty nasal spray bottle. Use 3 times daily to help unblock the nose and eustachian tubes, thus relieving the pressure and pain. If your child has a blocked nose, give the herbs horseradish and garlic. These will help clear the nose and sinuses and reduce pressure and pain.

Eczema (see Dermatitis)

Epilepsy

Epilepsy is not a disease in itself. It is an abnormal brain function in which there is a change in the nerve function of the brain caused by an abnormal electrical activity. It is this abnormality that causes a seizure or 'fit'. These seizures may recur at intervals of months or minutes. Seizures may be caused by a tumour, heavy drinking, withdrawal from anti-convulsant drugs, injury, infection or damage before birth or at birth, but more commonly there is no definable cause.

Epileptic seizures which occur before a child is 2 years are usually caused by a birth defect, or a metabolic disease. From 2 to the age of 19 it is usually caused by febrile thrombosis, congenital birth injury, head injury, or infection such as meningitis. From 20 years of age, the cause is more likely to be brain neoplasm, head injury or stroke.

The most common names given to epileptic seizures are the *grand mal* and *petit mal*. However, they are more properly included in the following groups: partial or focal, including simple and complex partial; generalised including absence (*petit mal*) myoclonic, clonic or clonic tonic (*grand mal*) and atonic;

also continual (*status epilepticus*).. In this condition there is not a complete recovery between attacks which may be partial or generalised. The *grand mal* can be preceded by an aura or personal warning (which can last up to one minute) in the form of a smell, physical sensation, mental images, or strange thoughts. The sufferer may start to gurgle, jerk, twitch, and then convulse for several minutes. Loss of bladder and bowel control is possible. The person might drool and the lips might turn blue.

A *petit mal* may go unnoticed as the child may stare, twitch, blink and nod in a 5 to 30 second lapse in consciousness. Others may attribute this to a loss of attention which could affect the child's school life. This condition rarely affects adults.

Diagnosis: differentiating between partial or focal seizures and generalised seizures is of great importance to your doctor. If you witness a seizure, take notes and report to a medical practitioner exactly what happened. How the patient reacted is assessed through an electroencephalograph (EEG), skull X-rays, CAT scans, lumbar puncture, or an analysis of serum glucose and calcium levels. Diagnosis is important as the patient may be in danger if a seizure happens at work or play.

A variety of drugs is available - Dilantin, Mysoline, and Zarotin. Naturopathic medicine has also had positive results. Vitamin E has been shown to reduce the number of seizures. Some patients treated with vitamin E at Westmead Hospital showed a reduced number of seizures. However, not all found vitamin E of use. Other trials overseas found vitamin E of benefit for some patients.

Scullcap is an anti-convulsive herb. Used in combination with hops and passion flower, it was an ancient treatment for epilepsy. Scullcap is mentioned in the *British Herbal Pharmacopoeia* specifically for epilepsy.

Recent research has found that a Chinese formula which included *Scutellaria laterifolia* demonstrated dramatic therapeutic effects on unsuccessfully treated patients on standard allopathic anti-convulsive drugs. More evaluation of this treatment is needed.

Tests on epileptic children show that many have lower

magnesium, manganese and zinc concentrations in the blood than non-epileptics. Supplementation of these minerals is believed to help. Adding amino acids, taurine and a compound called dimethyl glycine to the diet may also be beneficial.

Diet is also important. Exclude from the diet all refined carbohydrates and any foods that have an adverse effect. Epilepsy must be managed by a medical practitioner. Do not discontinue medication unless advised by a medical practitioner.

SUPPLEMENTS

vitamin E	500iu daily with food
scullcap	500 to 1,000mg with food 3 times daily
magnesium phosphate	200mg 3 times daily
zinc	25mg daily with food
vitamin B6	50mg up to 3 times daily

Eyes and eyesight
Caffeine and eyesight
People who drink large amounts of coffee reduce the blood flow to the retina. Caffeinated soft drinks, tea and coffee are contra-indicated in people with eye problems and failing eyesight. It would be wise to reduce your consumption as they are related to cardiovascular disease and headaches.

Cataracts
As people grow older they can be affected by cataracts or clouding of the lens. Vision is affected and the eyes can have a watery look. The word comes from the Greek for 'falling water'.

The cause is not fully understood but it is believed that free radicals (see also IMMUNE SYSTEM) can be one of the causes. It is more common for cataracts to develop in elderly people. Research done in Canada found the taking of antioxidant nutrients (beta-carotene, vitamin E and C) reduced the occurrence. Eating leafy green vegetables and yellow vegetables is very important. However, the amounts needed to prevent cataracts are more than can be obtained from a normal diet. Supplementing the diet with antioxidants could be the best way.

Other conditions such as glaucoma, detached retina, exposure to X-rays and diabetes can also lead to the development of cataracts. It is very important to wear eye protection, such as sunglasses, wherever suitable. Modern surgery has advanced in the treatment of cataracts. The operation is simple and successful. In natural therapy it is prevention, not surgical cure, that is the focus. Blueberries are a food which helps prevent cataracts and they should be eaten every day.

Glaucoma

There is evidence that blueberries can ease intra-ocular pressure. This herb seems to be of great value in the treatment of many eye disorders. A study done in Great Britain also revealed that fish oil relieved intra-ocular pressure in rabbits. When the supplement was decreased the pressure increased and vice versa. The diet needs to contain omega-3 fatty acids, found in deep sea oily fish.

Night vision

Poor eyesight at night has been found to be the result of lack of beta-carotene and vitamin A. These are important nutrients for the production of visual purple needed for night vision. In our society computer screens, television and bright lights can damage the visual purple and damage our night vision. There is also considerable evidence that blueberries can improve night vision. Blueberries restore visual acuity after exposure to bright light (glare) and can improve vision in low light.

SUPPLEMENTS (for all of the above)
natural beta-carotene (provitamin A)	6mg daily with main meal
vitamin A	10,000 iu daily
vitamin C	1,000mg daily
vitamin E	500mg daily
(all above vitamins found in antioxidant formula)	
blueberry (bilberry)	100mg extract 3 times daily

fresh blueberry	2 - 4oz 3 times daily
cod liver oil	children 2.5ml daily
	adults 5ml daily

Fevers

A fever is a rise in body temperature above normal. Most children have a fever at one time or another. Most fevers are not serious and are part of the development process in strengthening the immune system. However, it is important to monitor fevers and if needed keep them under control. All households where a baby or young children reside should have a thermometer to measure a rise in body temperature.

NORMAL BODY TEMPERATURE
oral   36.1-37.1°C
rectal   36.6-37.8°C
armpit   35.6-36.6°C

A rise in body temperature above 37.1°C when the temperature is taken orally is a fever. This is not a cause for alarm as body temperature varies throughout the day. A fever is the body's way of fighting an illness and does not have to be treated unless the temperature is over 38.9°C. If the fever starts to rise beyond this level then sponging the child and fanning will help bring relief. Even temperatures of up to 41.5°C do not cause brain damage and young children may often have fevers with temperatures nearing this level without any after-effects.

Babies under 12 months of age are different and abnormally high or low temperatures should be discussed with a practitioner for proper assessment. Fever can be harmless and only an indicator of a disease. What is to be observed is the activity and appearance of the child. If it is advised that the fever should be brought down, sponging with water is one of the best methods.

Yarrow, peppermint and elderflower mixed in equal parts and drunk as a tea can help reduce fever. Do not let a fever persist for more than 24 hours.

Care should be taken in administering drugs to young children. Aspirin should not be used if the child is suffering from chickenpox or influenza. A serious complication called Reye's Syndrome may develop in a small number of cases.

SUPPLEMENTS

vitamin C	250mg daily just before food children over 12 years take one 1,000mg vitamin C tablet daily
garlic equivalent to 2,000mg	over 12 years of age take 1 tablet daily with food

Fish and fish liver oils

The use of fish oil and fish liver oil for the treatment of illness and the promotion of good health has for decades been a part of life for many of us. Our grandparents used cod liver oil to prevent and treat coughs, colds and bronchial complaints with excellent results. We now know that the use of fish oil has even greater benefits. It is now used successfully in the reduction of arthritic pain and the prevention of certain types of cardiovascular disease. Other research suggests that fish oil may help prevent certain types of cancer.

There are 2 types of fish oil that are commercially available. They are the oil obtained from the liver of the fish which is high in vitamins A and D, and the oil obtained from the flesh of the fish which is very low in these vitamins.

Cold-water, oily fish such as herrings, cod, mackerel, tuna, sardines and salmon are used for oil extraction. These fish contain relatively high levels of the omega-3 fatty acids eicosapentaenoic and docosahexaenoic acid. These fatty acids are normally broken down (desaturated) in our bodies from linolenic acid, a fatty acid found in animal fat. This may sound a little confusing but it simply means that if our bodies do not desaturate linoleic acid properly then we may need to obtain these fatty acids from a food source. The best source of these important fatty acids is fish oil.

Fatty acids are crucial components in membrane structures and play an important role in the circulation of blood cells. The benefits of fish oil were first realised when it was noticed that the Eskimos of Greenland and Canada who retained their traditional fish diet had a much lower incidence of chronic diseases including coronary heart disease than the Eskimos who had changed their eating habits to a high animal fat Western-type diet.

The main benefits that have been reported when using fish oil as a supplement are - a reduction in the levels of blood triglyceride (one of the fats in the blood), a decrease in blood viscosity (blood thickness) and the reduction of the blood's ability to form blood clots. The combination of these beneficial effects may account for the significant reduction in the incidence of heart disease among fish eaters.

Clinical studies carried out on healthy subjects, as well as on patients with either heart disease or high cholesterol, showed that supplementing the diet with 3,600mg of fish oil daily, given over a 2 year period, reduced episodes of pain from angina, as well as decreasing triglycerides, cholesterol and bleeding time.

I have been asked the question, 'If fish oil reduces bleeding time could this cause other problems?' It is the thinning of the blood and the reduction of bleeding time that may be one of fish oil's greatest attributes, but as with any substance, very large doses may cause problems. If one were to take 15,000mg or more of fish oil daily then this could lead to excessive reductions in bleeding time and may cause haemorrhage. An easy way to prevent problems is to follow the directions on the bottle. I have found that 3,000mg to 6,000mg of fish oil daily gives good results, with safety.

Fish oil has also been shown to be of benefit in the treatment of the pain of arthritis. Supplementation of the diet with eicosapentaenoic acid, an omega-3 fatty acid found in fish oil, significantly reduced the stiffness and tenderness of painful joints in arthritic sufferers.

Fish oil's anti-inflammatory and antibiotic-like properties have been well demonstrated in scientific research, and it is this action that may account for cod liver oil's positive results when used for the treatment of bronchitis, upper respiratory infections and asthma, now said to be an inflammatory disease.

Studies conducted in Australia by Professor Ann Woolcock found that eating fish could help prevent asthma. This was supported by a statement made by Dr Craig Mellis, from Camperdown Children's Hospital who said that Aboriginal children also had very low rates of asthma and those who lived traditional lifestyles in Cape York had the lowest rates of all.

Professor Woolcock said that families who live in areas with a high incidence of asthma should eat fish. Although our grandmothers may not have known why fish oils worked so well when used for the treatment of many complaints, the positive results that they achieved over so many years give us confidence in using this time proven remedy.

NOTE: If you feel you are a sufferer of cardiovascular disease, then see your practitioner for professional assessment and advice.

German measles (Rubella)

Rubella is a virus which is highly contagious. A person can catch rubella by being sneezed or coughed on by an infected person. It most commonly affects children and adolescents but can also affect adults. The first symptoms are aches and pains and a pink, spotted rash behind the ears, on the chest and limbs. The eyes and the lymph glands get very sore. Bed rest and lots of fluids are the only treatment usually needed for rubella. The itchiness of the rash can be relieved with calamine lotion or Stop Itch Formula (see also CHICKENPOX).

The greatest danger of rubella is to the unborn fetus. It can cause deafness and blindness, and damage to the brain and heart. The danger period is in the first 16 weeks of pregnancy. Pregnant women who have been exposed to rubella should see their medical practitioner as soon as possible.

The best way to treat the child is to keep him or her in a darkened room with one shaded light. Manage the fever (see also FEVER) and give plenty of water and warm broth to drink.

Headache

Children do get headaches and they should be examined by taking notice of the frequency, the location, which side of the head, whether local pain or general pain and when they appear. Also note if there are other symptoms such as vomiting. Child migraines come on suddenly with flashing lights and wavy lines in front of the eyes and throbbing. They are on one side of the head, and create severe pain.

Adolescents are prone to tension headaches especially around exam time or if they are having problems with parents. The pain starts in the back of the neck and is dull and throbbing, moving up to the temples. Sleep will usually clear the headache. Viruses and sinusitis also cause terrible headaches. If the headache is accompanied by fever, vomiting and stiff neck then a medical practitioner should be called because it is symptomatic of a more serious condition (see also ALLERGIES).

SUPPLEMENTS

valerian	as directed on bottle
white willow bark	as directed on bottle
feverfew	for migraine 50mg in morning for 6 years and over

Heartburn (see Indigestion)

Heart disease (see Immune system, Fish oil)

Hepatitis

There are 3 types of hepatitis — types A, B and the new type C. These are viral infections which cause an inflammation of the liver. Type A is the infectious one which is thought to be caught from contact with faeces via food, poor sanitation, not washing the hands after going to the toilet, polluted water, or seafood caught near an ocean outfall. If a child has been in contact with an infected person it is wise to take the precaution of having a preventative injection. The period of incubation is 2 to 7 weeks in which time the child will become irritable. The symptoms are malaise, loss of appetite, fatigue, vomiting, headaches and chills and fever. Jaundice will appear - the child will go yellow and the liver enlarge painfully.

Type B is harder to contract as it is transmitted through contaminated syringes or blood transfusions. It takes 7 to 26 weeks to develop. Symptoms are dark urine and pale stools, fever, jaundice, fatigue, weakness and drowsiness. Recovery is certain but the liver needs help and the process is slow.

The liver is the second largest organ in the body and it produces and stores glycogen which is made from glucose and used by the muscles for energy. It produces bile which breaks down fats in the body and is important in the absorption of vitamin K from the intestines. It manufactures cholesterol which aids in the production of bile salts and steroid hormones. Drugs and chemicals are broken down in the liver and detoxified, including the body's own adrenalin which is recycled through the liver. It stores vitamins A, B12 and D, iron and copper, to feed the body. It forms new blood cells, destroys old red cells and 'throws them out', makes the protein in blood plasma, and produces the clotting agents in the blood.

Hepatitis inflames the liver and slows its functioning. If this happens, the liver, which normally helps remove toxins, stops work and the toxins build up in other organs, such as the skin, causing dermatitis and acne. The liver responds well to herbal treatment. Dandelion and milk thistle act as cholagogues. Dandelion has been said to be able to dissolve gallstones. Boldo is another powerful herb for the restoration of liver health. The vitamin B group is vital to liver health as is vitamin A. All these supplements are available for children and will be far more potent in a child recovering from hepatitis. Clinical studies have shown that *Sylibum marianum* helps reduce damage to the liver by some infections and toxins. This herb is therefore invaluable in the treatment of hepatitis.

SUPPLEMENTS
Sylibum marianum   1ml of 1:1 extract 3 times daily

dandelion tea	3 cups daily
zinc	1 tablet daily
multi B formula	
(sustained release)	1 tablet daily
sodium sulphate	3 times daily

Hernia

A hernia is ruptured tissue sticking out through an opening in whatever normally confines it, such as part of the intestine protruding through the muscular wall of the abdomen. This is the common type of hernia men and women get from lifting heavy objects.

Children most commonly suffer from inguinal or groin hernias and umbilical hernia which is a bulge beneath the area where the umbilical cord was attached. Sometimes reaching the size of an orange these types of hernias are more common in girls than in boys. Umbilical hernias usually recede by the time the child is 1 or 2 years and do not need any treatment.

Groin hernias are seen as a bulge alongside the penis or in the scrotum in boys and with girls in the groin area. Groin hernias can incarcerate (be unable to retract). If this happens the child will suffer pain and be irritable. The bowel, or the blood supply to the bowel, may become restricted resulting in strangulation of the area. This is a medical emergency. See your practitioner or take your child to hospital.

Herpes (see Cold sores)

Hiccups

Hiccups are an irritation of the nerves of the diaphragm caused by inhaling too much air, drinking carbonated liquids, gulping down food, eating chillies, drinking too much alcohol or even from laughing.

Babies get hiccups from gulping air when breastfeeding. It's important to burp baby regularly as excessive wind will cause the stomach to distend causing hiccups, wind pain and colic. Dill water will settle this colic.

A safe and certain solution for hiccups is raspberry syrup. It usually stops hiccups immediately. Use only raspberry juice and raw sugar, not low cal or artificially coloured and flavoured cordial.

DOSAGE

Raspberry juice	1 to 6 months 2.5 - 5ml
	6 to 12 months 5 -10ml
	12 months and over
	10 -20ml

Hives (Urticaria)

This is a common complaint with children. They break out in red, itchy swellings on the skin. The most common cause is allergy. This can be a reaction to anything from sugar to a plant. The histamines run freely through the body and fluid accumulates in the skin and mucous membranes. Cold compresses relieve the pain and swelling (see also DERMATITIS).

SUPPLEMENTS

vitamin C	6 to 12 years 1,000mg daily
	12 and over 2,000mg daily
ephedra	as directed by medical practitioner
zinc cream	as directed

(See also DERMATITIS and ECZEMA for formula)

Hormone Replacement Therapy

Every woman experiences menopause (see also OSTEOPOROSIS), or change of life, between the ages of 40 and 60. The side effects can be devastating, ranging from hot flushes to bad temper and depression.

As oestrogen levels decrease during and after menopause, calcium in the body is leached from the bones into the blood. The result for many women is a weakening of the bones and the onset of the disease osteoporosis. Dowager's hump and brittle bones which break easily are two results.

Quite often hormone replacement therapy from your medical practitioner is recommended and can be the answer but there are other options. The Chinese have used hormone replacement therapy in the form of herbs for thousands of years. An example of the power of herbs is the fact that the Aztec Indians used herbs for contaception thousands of years ago. The Chinese have used dong quai for many female problems including menopause. Dong quai contains plant oestrogens or phyto-oestrogens and it is an adapting or adaptogenic herb. When the body's oestrogen level is low, it adds to the oestrogen in the body, increasing circulating oestrogen. When the oestrogen levels are high it competes for the binding sites reducing the effect of oestrogen. Dong quai will reduce hot flushes and calcium loss.

Evening primrose oil is of advantage to many women. The essential fatty acids in the oil have hormone balancing properties due to their action on the prostaglandin pathway. Women suffering from depression during menopause should eat whole rolled oats (avena) or take an oat supplement. Oats help balance the fluctuations of moods during menopause as they are an effective antidepressant and are also nutritious and beneficial for good health. Menopause is not unlike pre-menstrual tension (see PMT). Supplementing with a B group vitamin will help through the menopausal changes.

Bone fractures can be reduced by taking fish oil. Vitamin D or pre-formed vitamin D found in cod liver oil for instance, seems to prevent osteomalacia. This is one of the causes of bone fractures. Studies indicate that people supplementing with fish oil, extra calcium and multi vitamin and mineral formula, reduce the incidence of osteoporosis and osteomalacia. I recommend about a teaspoon of cod liver oil a day. This will avoid overdosing on vitamin A and D. If you are eating a lot of kidney or liver then you probably do not need this much. Do not rely on offal as your source of these vitamins as the toxins built up in these organs can cause a build up in similar organs in your own body.

It is vital to reduce the chance of weakening bones and osteoporosis. Regular exercise, 30 minutes walking 4 times a week, will help strengthen bones. Bones can actually grow with exercise, even after menopause has taken place. Calcium is also critical to the diet. Between 800 and 1,200 mg a day is required. A combination of the above is a natural way of approaching menopause, and will help relieve the symptoms and resulting conditions. Try the natural way before you experiment with heavier medication.

SUPPLEMENTS

dong quai	500mg dried herb morning and night
evening primrose oil	2 to 4 capsules of 500mg daily
cod liver oil	4mls daily
vitamin D	only if not taking cod liver oil
calcium	1,000mg daily

Hyperactivity

As parents tear their hair out and the child screams around the house, everyone is asking the question, 'What's wrong?' The child is far more active than a child of that age should be. They are loud, noisy, squirm, run about, teachers complain and babysitters will not sit. When you go to their room in the morning the sheets are in a tangled mass on the floor (see also HYPOGLYCAEMIA).

Although some theorists think hyperactivity is hereditary, most believe it is related to diet — too much sugar and food containing artificial dyes and additives, and refined carbohydrates are known causes of hyperactivity. Your child could possibly be allergic to salycilates (see also ALLERGIES). To find out which food causes problems, restrict suspected foods from the diet for a few weeks then re-introduce them, one at a time. If the problem returns, then restrict the food for at least 3 months before trying it again.

A herbal mixture which will calm your child down is Nervaid which contains the herbs scullcap, passiflora, hops and valerian, in combination. To work out the child's dosage, divide their age by their age + 12, for example if the child is 6 divide 6 by 6 + 12 = 18 = .33. The child takes 33 per cent of the adult dose.

SUPPLEMENTS

herbal nerve formula	as directed
child multi vitamin	1 tablet daily
Magnesium complex	6 to 12 years 1 tablet 3 times daily
Nervaid	6 to 12 years 1 tablet morning and night

Hypoglycaemia (Low blood sugar)

When the blood sugar (glucose) is at a level below that needed for normal bodily function, it can affect not only good health but also behaviour. Children who are hypoglycaemic often have one or more of the following symptoms - nervousness, cold sweats, weakness, a feeling of fatigue and irritability, confusion, unusual behaviour, and in extreme cases such as insulin dependent diabetes, unconsciousness can occur. All of the above symptoms can be relieved by taking sugar. However, the process repeats itself and the symptoms return. Sufferers of diabetes must see their medical practitioner for treatment and a child who is a diabetic and suffers a 'hypo' must be given sugar urgently.

Low blood sugar is very often traced to poor diet and an excessive consumption of refined carbohydrates over too long a period. A high sugar diet worsens the condition by increasing the demand for insulin (the hormone needed to utilise glucose within the body). As the blood insulin increases, the sugar level falls, and if too much insulin is produced then it lowers the body's glucose level and aggravates the condition. Eating more sugar only temporarily relieves the condition because the insulin levels soon rise and down falls the blood sugar level.

Changing the diet is the only way of changing the condition and helping to prevent the possible onset of diabetes mellitus later in life. A diet low in refined carbohydrates and fat and higher in protein and complex carbohydrates will, over a period, return blood sugar levels to normal.

Children with mild episodes respond to orange juice, honey and dried fruits. Clinical studies have found that supplementing with the mineral chromium, found in GTF (glucose tolerance factor) chromium yeast, can alleviate the symptoms of hypoglycaemia within 3 months. The mineral magnesium may help reduce glucose induced insulin secretion.

SUPPLEMENTS.

magnesium phosphate compound	children over 6 years 1 tablet 3 times daily
GTF chromium yeast	1 tablet twice daily

Hypothermia

It is unusual for children to suffer hypothermia in Australia unless they have been exposed to cold winds and water. During hypothermia the body temperature drops below the norm, pulse and breathing slows, the child or adult may be confused and tired and, if not treated properly and quickly, may die.

If possible, move the victim out of the elements, away from cold winds and damp. Warm them so the temperature rises gradually, using two blankets lying on top of each other, and your own body stripped to give more direct warmth. Under no circumstances use heaters, fire, alcohol or massage to warm the person. This can cause a rush of blood to the skin which can result in a sudden drop in body core temperature, worsening the condition. If the person is conscious, give them sips of warm sweet drinks or soup.

Immune system
and cardiovascular disease

Viral infections and suppressed immune systems are becoming a greater problem today than they were 20 years ago. Diseases such as Acquired Immune Deficiency Syndrome (AIDS), Chronic Fatigue Syndrome and viral infections, are presenting practitioners and the public with symptoms not previously encountered.

When we take a closer look at the empirical use of herbal medicine, we note that the active constituents of herbs were not known to ancient herbalists, and it was probably trial and error through the centuries that eventually led to the specific use of certain herbs in the treatment of specific ailments. Even today, many of the active principles of herbs are still unknown and the reliance on empirical evidence is still our main scientific justification for using these herbs.

Garlic One of the most common herbs used by the ancients and indeed modern herbalists, for the treatment of infection is *Allium sativum* (garlic). Garlic is a member of the lily family and it contains a volatile oil composed of compounds which contain sulphur : allicin, diallyl disulfide, diallyl trisulfide and others.

Garlic was used for the treatment of amoebic dysentery by Albert Schweitzer in Africa and its antibiotic activity was first noted by Louis Pasteur. Garlic's antiseptic action was used in the prevention of gangrene during the first and second world wars. Herbalists are now using garlic either in combination with other herbs or by itself in the treatment of the common cold, sinusitis and upper respiratory tract infections and in fact, garlic is mentioned in the *British Herbal Pharmacopoeia* for the treatment of these conditions.

Unfortunately, garlic has a very pungent odour and investigations have shown that the allicin in garlic is the ingredient responsible for this odour. Research shows that allicin could be the major active constituent in garlic that inhibits the growth of Staphyloccus, Streptococcus, Bacillus, Brucella and Vibrio species at low concentrations. This would suggest that deodorised garlic may not be as efficacious.

Garlic's anti-viral effects have also been demonstrated *in vivo*. Garlic was shown to protect mice infected with influenza virus from infections. It also enhanced the neutralising antibody production when given with influenza vaccine.

Many *in vitro* and *in vivo* studies have been carried out demonstrating garlic's effect on influenza B, herpes simplex,

Coxsackie virus, Rhinovirus and *Candida albicans*.

Echinacea *Echinacea angustifolia's* use as an anti-viral herb which stimulates the immune system is well documented. It is the extracts from the root of the purple coneflower which possess properties which stimulate immunity to viruses. This is probably due to its polysaccharide components. These polysaccharides bind themselves to the activated carbohydrate receptors of the T-lymphocytes.

This action results in the production of interferon and enhances natural killer cell activity.

This result leads to destruction of the invading virus and an increase in the number of T-lymphocytes, making echinacea an ideal herb to consider for diseases such as influenza and post-viral syndrome.

Beta-carotene Although there are several hundred carotenoids in the food chain which are found in leafy green and yellow vegetables, the most abundant that humans can metabolise to retinol (vitamin A) is the carotenoid, beta-carotene.

Research has found that beta-carotene, along with some other carotenoids, shows enhancement of immune responsiveness and reduction of induced nuclear damage. Low levels of beta-carotene in serum or plasma are consistently associated with the subsequent development of lung cancer.

Other new research world-wide has found that increased levels of beta-carotene in the diet reduce the risk of coronary heart disease and cancer. One Australian study found that patients given 20mg of beta-carotene daily for 12 months improved their blood lipid profile by increasing the HDL level.

Further evidence of the benefits of supplementing with beta-carotene was highlighted by a study conducted at the Harvard Medical School, USA. In this study which involved 22,000 male doctors, it was found that men who already suffer from ischaemic heart disease and who supplemented their diets with beta-carotene, had 50 per cent less heart attacks and strokes than those who were not taking supplements.

At the annual conference of the Nutritional Society of Australia, Dr Meyskens, head of the Clinical Cancer Centre at the University of California, Irvine, said there is substantial scientific evidence linking beta-carotene with low rates of lung and breast cancer and heart disease.

Vitamin C has probably been considered by most people when looking for a natural way of treating the common cold. The reason for their choice was mostly based on the work carried out by Professor Linus Pauling. Many people have said that Linus Pauling's work has not been vindicated in recent trials. However, I do not believe this to be true. Recent double-blind trials on vitamin C have shown that the symptoms of the common cold can be dramatically reduced by taking 2,000mg of vitamin C daily. It is probable that ascorbic acid assists the immune system and acts against pathogens, especially bacteria and viruses.

Based on the ascorbic acid content of a primitive vegetarian diet, Pauling estimated that modern people need a diet with an average of 2.3g of vitamin C per day. The degree of supplementation required will, of course, depend on individual diet and lifestyle, but 2.3g of vitamin C per day will lead to an ascorbic acid blood concentration about 3 times the unsupplemented level. Tobacco smoking lowers serum vitamin C (each cigarette destroys about 25mg of ascorbic acid), and some smokers suffer from chronic, sub-clinical scurvy.

Nitrosamines, formed from dietary amines and nitrite (present in preserved food or produced naturally from nitrate), are perhaps the most universal and potent class of carcinogen. We are exposed to them continuously, and they are probably the specific cause of gastric (stomach) cancer. Several are present in tobacco and tobacco smoke. Ascorbic acid destroys nitrosamines rapidly and completely, and a combination of vitamins C and E is even more effective. A high concentration of free vitamin C in the stomach, intestines, bladder and tissues would seem to be desirable for protection against nitrosamines.

The argument is often put forward that intakes of vitamin C greater than about 150mg per day are unnecessary because, when more than this is taken, vitamin C often appears in the urine. However, despite its appearance in the urine, much more than 150mg per day is usually needed to ensure tissue saturation of the vitamin. There are no known ill effects of vitamin C when taken at the rate of 1 to 3 grams per day. The frequently raised connection between oxalate renal (kidney) stones and vitamin C is false, and arose from inadequate analytical methods, where urinary vitamin C interfered in the determination of oxalate.

Further benefits of vitamin C were noted following an epidemiological study of 11,348 adults conducted by the University of California which found that men who consumed the most vitamin C had a 42 per cent lower death rate from all causes than men in the lower intake group, and could expect to live 6 to 7 years longer. Hardening of the arteries, a major cause of death from heart disease, nearly stopped in those patients who supplemented with the antioxidants beta-carotene, vitamin C and vitamin E.

Vitamin E (d-alpha-tocopherol) is a powerful antioxidant and has been the subject of much research. Back in the 1950s, Drs W. and E. Shute of Canada first published papers on the use of vitamin E in the treatment of cardiovascular disease. Recent studies have given further credence to their findings and a recent case controlled study published in the *Lancet* which involved 110 cases suffering from angina and 394 controls, showed an inverse correlation between vitamin E intake and the risk of suffering angina.

Several medical uses of vitamin E have been developed based on an increased understanding of the damaging effects of free radical induced events in tissues. Oxidant species, especially those produced by lipid peroxidation, appear to contribute to the etiology and pathology of chronic diseases including cataract, cardiovascular disease, emphysema, reperfusion injury, and rheumatoid arthritis, as well as cancer. As the body's principal lipid-soluble antioxidant, vitamin E may play an important role in the amelioration and treatment of these and other disorders.

It appears that antioxidant supplementation slows down the oxidation of low density lipoprotein (LDL) which has a direct effect on atherosclerosis.

The results we have gained in the treatment of many viral

and virus related illnesses have been extremely good. The most common would be patients presenting with influenza or common colds, and although full double-blind trials have not been carried out, our patient trials have demonstrated dramatic improvement in all symptoms of these viral infections when taking this combination.

I have also used this combination of herbs and nutrients when treating patients suffering from post-viral syndrome and those who are constantly contracting viral infections. The results of these studies have show a marked improvement in the patients' resistance to infection.

I believe it is the combination of the anti-viral properties of echinacea and garlic, combined with the immune stimulating properties of the antioxidants, that enables us to successfully manage viral infections. Also, with the new positive research concerning antioxidants and their role in the prevention of disease, including cancer and heart disease, they are a must for inclusion in preventative medicine.

Impetigo (School sores)

Impetigo is the correct name for 'school sores'. To a parent it is horror when their child develops these festering sores which are contagious. Children with impetigo should be kept home from school while the sores are weeping and encouraged not to have close contact with other children.

Impetigo can first manifest in puffy patches on the face, scalp, neck, knees and elbows, and soon turn into blisters or pustules which then form crusts. However, these sores are mostly seen on the legs. The disease is caught by infection entering a break in the skin and then spread by scratching.

In the 1930s medicine thought these sores were cold sores and the name for impetigo then was also contagious cold sore (*impetigo contagiosa*). This is now known to be the result of a streptococcus or staphylococcus infection.

The medical treatment for impetigo is antibiotics. Unfortunately because of the overuse of some antibiotics, the staphylococcal infection that can cause impetigo is now resistant to many of them. Antibiotics may be needed but usually the natural medication works well.

The treatment for impetigo is simple and usually effective. The crusts on all sores must be removed. This can be done easily by washing the sore with a warm boric acid solution. To make this solution add 1 heaped teaspoon of boric acid powder to 600ml of boiling water, cool and then use. Once the sore is exposed, apply tea tree oil, or golden seal antiseptic ointment to the area, then cover with a sterile dressing. Do this twice daily. As with all infections, supplementing with herbs and nutrients that strengthen the immune system can be of great help.

SUPPLEMENTS

echinacea	children 6 to 12 years of age 1 tablet containing 175mg of the herb twice daily with food over 12 years 1 tablet 3 times daily
vitamin C	children 6 to 12 years chew a citrus C 250mg daily just before food children over 12 years take one 1,000mg vitamin C tablet daily
garlic	over 12 years of age take 1 enteric coated tablet equal to 2,000mg of fresh herb daily with food

Indigestion

This disorder is not a specific ailment as the symptoms can be due to gastro-intestinal disorders of various kinds. Usually an unhealthy lifestyle causes the body to cry out. Overeating is a common cause of indigestion and, in our society many people fall victim. Overeating will cause the stomach to become over-stretched and the natural motions of digestion will slow down. Also overeating causes other problems including obesity. Another common cause of indigestion is eating too quickly or washing food down with drink. This way of eating is very common with teenagers who just can't seem to get their food consumed quickly enough. Eating too quickly also causes gulping of air which all too often leads to bloating, discomfort and flatulence. Not chewing food properly prevents the correct stimulation of digestive enzymes. One of these, amylase, is formed by the saliva glands and is needed for the correct digestion of carbohydrate. It is important that your children's teeth be kept healthy as poor teeth can also lead to improper chewing and poor digestion.

Symptoms of indigestion can include nausea, biliousness, headaches, heartburn, lassitude and flatulence. Heartburn is caused by the stomach acids rising up into the food pipe (oesophagus) and then burning the sensitive lining. The herb slippery elm chewed just after meals will quickly bring relief. Slippery elm bark has soothing effects on the digestive tract and can ease the discomfort of ulcers in adults. Flatulence and colic are immediately eased by taking peppermint, slippery elm and charcoal which will absorb the toxins and gases which cause pain and wind.

Diet is important and should consist of three or four well-spaced meals a day which are nutritious and well-balanced, containing plenty of roughage, fresh fruit and vegetables. Seventy per cent of the energy intake from food should be from complex carbohydrates, 10 - 15 per cent should be from protein and 15 - 20 per cent from fat.

Digestive upset can also occur following antibiotic therapy; certain antibiotics, including tetracycline, although helping to control infection, can also kill off the friendly gut flora. If you or your child have been on antibiotics then include yoghurt in the diet the following week. Certain brands of yoghurt contain *Lactobacillus acidophilus*, the friendly bacteria needed for proper digestion of food. A supplement containing acidophilus can also be of great help in restoring the natural balance in the gastrointestinal tract.

SUPPLEMENTS

acidophilus and bifidus — children 6 to 12 years 2
(this formula relieves most — capsules with food

symptoms of indigestion)	twice daily
peppermint tea	3 cups daily
slippery elm	3 to 6 years 300mg twice daily just before food
Digestive Aid	12 years and over 1 tablet before food 3 times daily
Acid Eze	follow directions on tin

Lice

Head lice are far more common among children than you may think. Dirtiness is not the cause of lice. However, lice are more common or likely to be caught if the clothes and hair is not kept clean. Coming into contact with a child or object that is infested with lice is the cause. Most schools report an outbreak each year.

The lice suck blood from the skin causing redness and itchiness, the child often scratches the infested area and bacterial infection can develop. On close inspection of the hair, white eggs (nits) can be seen attached to individual strands. These eggs are small grey bodies that stick to the hair and cannot be brushed off easily.

If any member of the family becomes infested with lice then the whole family should be inspected. All the child's clothing should be treated along with combs, bedding and towels. Utensils including combs and hairbrushes should all be boiled and clothing either boiled or dry cleaned.

The child's hair should be washed thoroughly with a medicated shampoo with a few drops of tea tree oil added. Then, using a fine comb that has been dipped in vinegar, comb the hair from the roots one segment at a time to remove all the nits. Take your time as all nits need to be removed.

Menstruation

Menstruation, or periods, indicates a coming to womanhood for a young girl and should be seen as a positive and normal part of life. It is important to talk to your child before she starts her monthly menstrual cycle and inform her of all the changes that will occur to her body as she enters puberty.

The menstrual cycle is divided into 4 phases. Menstruation is the shedding of the endometrium and uterine bleeding. The proliferative phase is the stage when the uterine lining (epithelium) returns to normal. Also during this phase the ovarian follicle is secreting oestrogens. The luteal phase is the time in the period the ovary is secreting progesterone. This lasts for around 1 to 2 weeks. The final phase in the menstrual cycle is the premenstrual phase when small parts of dead endometrium tissue break away with menstrual fluid and the menstrual cycle begins.

Most young girls start their periods at the age of 12 to 13 years but they can start as early as 9 or as late as 16 years of age. You should explain to your daughter that her periods may take several months before her menstrual cycle becomes regular and this is not a cause of concern. The cycle ranges from 21 to 33 days with only a third of women having the classic 28 day cycle. Average bleeding is 5 days with some girls having a 1 day period and others a 9 day period. By far the majority of women report some forewarning of the period in the form of mood swings, bloating, water retention, soreness of the breasts, pimples, and abdominal pain. This is sometimes described as Premenstrual Tension (see PMT) and this experience is annoying and unpleasant for many women. This condition can be eased by taking evening primrose oil and the B group of vitamins.

A lack of zinc in the diet can cause slow sexual development and delay the onset of the menses. Ensure that the diet is rich in foods containing zinc: eggs, whole grains and black strap molasses. The herbs *Vitex agnus-castus* and dong quai can help regulate the menstrual cycle.

SUPPLEMENTS

multi vitamin and mineral	1 tablet daily with food
bio zinc	over 12 years and adults 1 tablet daily
evening primrose oil	500mg with food twice daily

Motion sickness

Many people may experience travel sickness at some time in their lives. It is common for children to become nauseated in the back seat of the car, necessitating a stop every hour or so. The feeling is caused by the effects of irregular movements which cause the motion detectors in the inner ear to disagree with what the eyes see. In other words, the eyes, when looking at objects in the car, don't notice movement but the middle ear notices all movement. The different messages sent to the brain can cause nausea and vomiting.

A fishing, aeroplane, overseas or car trip can be spoilt by motion sickness in both children and adults. In the car it is effective to put the sick child near an open window, avoid reading or looking at objects in the car and look out at the scenery. Avoid greasy and junk foods, and always eat a wholesome breakfast as an empty stomach can make things worse. Clinical studies have found that the herb ginger is a very successful treatment that (unlike other anti-nausea medications) is without problematic side-effects. Peppermint is also calming to the digestive system and can help relieve nausea.

SUPPLEMENTS

Travel Calm Ginger	take 1 tablet 2 hours before trip and then 1 tablet every hour or as directed on bottle
peppermint tea	children over 3 years of age, drink 1 cup with the ginger just before the journey

Nappyrash

Babies commonly suffer nappy rash and this can be the result of being wet or a reaction to foods in the diet (see also ALLERGIES). If wet nappies are causing the problem, a powder of cornflour and zinc dusted on the rash will soothe it as will zinc cream or a moisture repellant jelly. Tea tree oil, diluted with glycerine will help kill the thrush and soothe the pain for the baby. Always dry baby properly and allow the little bottom to air without nappies as much as possible If the rash is caused by thrush or candida, then acidophilus in yoghurt will need to be added to the diet to help counteract the candida. Tea tree oil, diluted with glycerine will help kill the thrush and soothe the pain for the baby.

Nosebleed

This is one of the common afflictions of childhood. It is usually caused by the rupturing of blood vessels in the nose which is set off by such childish things as picking the nose, a bang on the nose or head, nose polyps or small growths, infections or allergic reactions which in turn create excessive sneezing. More extreme causes can include high blood pressure, heart disease, leukemia, and the clotting components of the blood. Frequent and severe bleeding must be referred to a medical practitioner.

Home treatment of the problem is to apply a cold compress of ice in a plastic bag, wrapped in a teatowel, applying pressure to the nose with the forefinger and thumb. Sit the child upright and lean forward slightly to prevent the blood running down the throat.

SUPPLEMENTS

vitamin C complex	contains 1,000mg of vitamin C and bioflavonoids (strengthen the capillaries and blood vessels)

Nutrition

The food we eat requires a complex action by the digestive system with the utilisation of enzymes to break down protein, carbohydrates and fats. In turn, the effectiveness of the process is affected by pollution, illness and stress. As a result, good health is diminished.

The importance of choosing foods that contain no artificial

colouring, flavouring or preservatives must be emphasised. These additives can cause allergies and digestive problems.

The 6 basic nutrients which make up our food are:
1. Water
2. Carbohydrates
3. Fats
4. Proteins
5. Vitamins
6. Minerals

Water makes up 70 per cent of our body and is needed to regulate the body's temperature, to form blood and body fluids to carry nutrients to the cells and to remove waste products. You must drink 6 to 8 glasses of water a day to keep joints, skin and organs young. It is also very important for the health of the brain.

Carbohydrates mainly function to supply the body with energy and for the formation of cellular constituents. A lack of carbohydrates will lead to an excess of ketones within the body. This excess of ketones increases the acidity of the blood resulting in a condition known as metabolic acidosis and this is a dangerous condition. Fad diets, including liquid high protein meal replacement foods, can cause this condition.

Carbohydrate intake should be 60 to 65 per cent of our total diet. Whole grains and potatoes are good sources of complex carbohydrates (polysaccharides) and are also good sources of fibre as are whole fruits and vegetables. Other carbohydrates include sugar, which is a disaccharide or double sugar, and glucose, which is a monosaccharide or single sugar. Avoid refined sugar from a packet. If you want sweetening on cereal, use whole fruits.

Fats are a very important part of the diet as they provide energy (twice as much as carbohydrates) and insulate the body, protecting it from sudden temperature change and damage.

Fats are made up of essential fatty acids. There are three: linoleic, linolenic and arachidonic. These fatty acids are essential and must become an integral part of our daily diet. It is best that our dietary intake of fats comes from the vegetable kingdom as these fats are unsaturated and include polyunsaturated fatty acids. Animal fats are high in saturated fatty acids and cholesterol and are associated with an increase in cardiovascular disease. The total energy intake derived from fats in the diet should be around 25 to 30 per cent.

Protein is needed for new growth, building cells and repairing tissues. It forms hormones and enzymes, important in growth, metabolism and sexual development. Proteins are made up of amino acids of which there are 22, 8 of which are essential and must be obtained from our food. They are the building blocks of protein and their distribution in foods determines whether the protein is complete or incomplete.

Complete proteins are foods that contain all the 8 essential amino acids; incomplete proteins do not contain them in any significant quantity. The mixing of complete and incomplete proteins in one meal is the best way of receiving a high quality protein meal and other micro nutrients needed for good health. The 8 essential amino acids are lysine, tryptophan, phenylalanine, methionine, threonine, leucine, isoleucine and valine.

Egg is the highest quality protein, followed by dairy products and meat. It is not necessary to consume large quantities of red meat to receive all the protein that our body requires to remain healthy. The energy intake from protein should be approximately 10 per cent of our total energy intake.

GRAMS OF PROTEIN NEEDED EACH DAY

Age in years	Per kg of ideal body weight
1 to 3	1.78
4 to 6	1.50
7 to 10	1.20
11 to 14	1.00
15 to 18	0.86
19 and over	0.80
pregnant women	1.36
lactating mothers	1.17
65 and over	1.10

It is easy to work out your ideal daily requirement of protein. Multiply your ideal body weight by the number of grams of protein. An adult whose ideal weight is 70kg would require 56gms of protein a day, i.e. 70 x 0.80 = 56 gms / day.

Vitamins help regulate the metabolism and assist in the release of energy from foods within the body. Vitamins also function as co-enzymes and catalysts. This action assists the chemical reactions that are continually taking place in a healthy body.

Vitamins are oil or water soluble. Water soluble vitamins are the B and C groups; oil includes the A, D, K and E groups. Water soluble vitamins are quickly utilised within the body and only remain in tissue for a short time, so they need to be replaced daily. Fat soluble vitamins last a lot longer and are stored in the liver or fatty tissue.

Minerals act as co-enzymes and are an important part of many metabolic processes. A deficiency of minerals in our diets can lead to illness. A lack of iron or calcium in the diet can cause anaemia or osteoporosis.

Recent research carried out by the Department of Health and Community Services found that a large number of Australians were not getting the recommended dietary intake (RDI) of vitamins and minerals. Zinc is one mineral deficient in the Australian diet. Of women, 83.4 per cent and of men, 52.9 per cent, aged between 35 and 44 were not getting the RDI of zinc in their diets. Zinc is an essential constituent of over 90 enzymes in our bodies and a deficiency can result in impaired growth and sexual development in the young. As we grow older, a lack of zinc in our diets can result in premature greying of the hair and the enlargement of the prostate gland in men.

Vitamin and mineral deficiencies in the Australian soil, and loss of them in overcooking food, are two reasons for inadequacies in our diets. Food storage may cause a reduction in the nutritional value as does gas ripening of fruit and vegetables. There is often a long period between the harvesting of food and the arrival on the table for consumption.

Poor digestion, alcohol, laxatives, smoking, food storage,

fad diets, prescription drugs and antibiotics, the contraceptive pill, ageing, overexercising and poor diet are all reasons for supplementation with vitamins and minerals.

Digestion is important to the absorption of food. Eat only natural foods. Avoid artificial colourings, flavourings and preservatives. Eat raw foods whenever possible. Make 80 per cent of your food alkaline. Do not eat and drink at the same time and take time to eat your meals. Plan when and where you are going to eat your next meal and sit down and enjoy it. It will make you think more about what you are eating. Spice up your food with garlic, lemon, vinegar and oil rather than salt. Salt will harden your arteries and give you high blood pressure.

Acid and alkaline foods are defined by the amount of food residue, or ash, they leave in the body. An excess of alkaline food residue is what the body requires for good health. Our diets should contain 80 per cent of alkaline ash residue foods. These foods include all fruit and vegetables, soy beans and buckwheat. Grapefruit is one of the most alkaline fruits we can eat so remember taste is not an indicator. Acid foods should make up the other 20 per cent of the diet.

Most of the complete protein foods are acid forming: meat, eggs, whole wheat, nuts and cheese. If you eat large amounts of these acid foods, it can lead to heart disease, arthritis and metabolic acidosis.

Neutral residue foods include milk, butter and cold pressed vegetable oils. Neutral foods can be eaten freely but don't forget fat, carbohydrates and protein must be balanced. We need to eat a well-balanced diet obtained from a variety of foods. Try eating a different cereal each day and extend the range of vegetables, lean meats and fruit used in the preparation of other meals. As nutritional insurance, take a sustained release multi vitamin and mineral tablet each day.

Osteoporosis

A change in the hormonal pattern (see also HORMONE REPLACEMENT THERAPY) after menopause accelerates this disease in women. Osteoporosis is the leaching of calcium from the bones which begins around 30 years of age. To help prevent it women should supplement their diet with calcium phosphate and foods containing calcium. Dairy products and fish are very important foods to include in the diet all through a woman's life.

The diet should contain foods with a high alkaline ash residue, as found in fruit and vegetables. Foods with a high acid ash residue, such as meat, eggs, cereals and starches increase calcium and bone loss. As you grow older you should decrease protein and increase green, leafy vegetables in your diet.

Research has shown caffeine, nicotine and alcohol all accelerate loss of bone mass. Increasing the size and strength of bones can be accomplished with gentle exercise. You do not have to jog. Walking is fine. So is swimming. Tests done on dancers found their bones were growing, even when examined after menopause.

SUPPLEMENTS

calcium phosphate	2,000mg daily
vitamin D	400mg daily
folic acid	5mg daily
magnesium phosphate	100mg 3 times daily
multi vitamin mineral	1tablet daily

Parkinson's disease

Parkinson's disease is a degenerative disease that affects the nervous system. It is thought to be a result of an imbalance of the brain chemicals acetylcholine and dopamine. Although the cause is unknown, a deficiency of the chemical that helps the transfer of messages between nerve cells has been identified in certain cells.

Parkinson's disease was named after the British medical practitioner Dr James Parkinson. In the 1800s the disease, which he called 'shaking palsy', was treated by practitioners with blood letting and laxatives. This type of treatment is no longer used in medicine.

Early symptoms of Parkinson's disease include infrequent blinking and it progresses to include shuffling walk, tremors, loss of appetite, fixed facial expression and drooling. Tremor may be absent in about 30 per cent of patients in the early stages of the disease; tremor by itself may be essential tremor and not Parkinson's disease.

Herbal medicine was the only successful treatment for this condition in the past and until the introduction of L-dopa in the 1960s the herb deadly nightshade was the main medication prescribed to help control tremor. Other members of the Solanaceae family have also been used to treat the tremors associated with old age and Parkinson's disease. However, deadly nightshade has been the most useful, in particular the roots.

This works indirectly on the parasympathetic nervous system by preventing acetylcholine from exerting its usual action on receptor cells. This action helps control micturition, tremor and excessive production of saliva. Most studies were carried out using synthetic atropine as an adjunct therapy to levodopa and not the root extract of belladonna. More studies with regard to the use of the whole herb preparation of the root need to be undertaken.

The plant *Datura stramonium*, another in the Solanaceae family, is also of use in the control of sialorrhea (excessive flow of saliva), rigidity and tremor. Datura contains the alkaloids hyoscyamine, hyoscine and small amounts of atropine. *Datura stramonium* has also been used with good results in the treatment of asthma in particular when combined with lobelia and ephedra. Take 100mg 3 times daily of *Datura stramonium* (dried herb). This herb can only be medically supplied.

Ergot of rye (*Claviceps purpurea*) is a fungus that forms in the ovary of the rye plant. The eating of this fungus found on rye and other similar grasses in overdose caused a disease in humans called St Anthony's Fire. This disease was characterised by hallucination and madness. Ergot's use dates back to the fifteenth century when it was used for treatment in obstetrics. This was reported by the German herbalist, Lonitzer. This herb was also used in neurology. Ergot alkaloids are also used medically in the treatment of Parkinson's disease. They possess an antiparkinsonian activity by directly activating dopamine receptors in the brain. One of the alkaloid derivatives of ergot is bromocriptine. However, the use of this drug and other ergot alkaloids is limited because of a number of side effects including hypertension and delirium. Because of their toxicity, ergot alkaloids are now only used by medical practitioners.

Three other herbs that are of benefit when used for the treatment of tremor, rigidity and gait are scullcap, passion flower and valerian. These nervine herbs have anti-convulsive, anti-spasmodic and sedative properties that also seem to help not only the symptoms of the disease but also the general nervous system.

SUPPLEMENTS

scullcap	1,000mg dried herb with food 3 times daily
passion flower	500mg dried herb 3 times daily with food
valerian	500mg dried herb 3 times daily with food

Caution using vitamin B6

Care should be taken by patients who have been medically prescribed levodopa because vitamin B6 may counteract the effects of this drug. This is because levodopa, a dopaminergic agent that converts into dopamine in the body, unlike dopamine when taken orally, can cross the brain blood barrier thus increasing dopamine levels in the brain. The following foods are high in vitamin B6 and should be avoided or consumed in moderation only: bananas, whole grains, fish, organ meats, red meat, peanuts, potatoes and oatmeal.

The sufferer should be placed on a low protein diet and only eat one small protein meal daily at night and not with medication. Digested protein prevents the absorption and utilisation of medication. Studies have shown that a low protein diet allows a reduction in the dosage of L-dopa and at the same time discontinuance of some of the medication needed to control the side effects of the drug. The diet should consist of 75 per cent raw foods including fruits and vegetables but limit the foods mentioned previously if taking medication. Avoid excessive exposure to manganese, as this is associated with increased risk of parkinsonism. Brain dopamine production depends on vitamin B6; studies have also found that supplementation may help decrease cramps, trembling and rigidity. The drug most often medically prescribed for this disease is levodopa. DO NOT take vitamin B6 (Pyridoxine) with this medication as it may counteract the effects of this drug.

OTHER SUPPLEMENTS

vitamin B6	100mg daily (not if on L-dopa)
vitamin B1	100mg daily may help rigidity
evening primrose oil	500mg with food 3 times daily
calcium phosphate	1,000mg elemental calcium daily (for nerve impulse transmission)
magnesium phosphate	130mg twice daily (for nerve impulse transmission)

The use of **amino acids** can be of great assistance in managing the symptoms of the disease. Studies have found that supplementation with D-phenylalanine may improve speech difficulties, depression and rigidity.

DOSAGE:
D-phenylalanine 250mg twice daily (not with meals) for speech difficulties, depression and rigidity
L-methionine 500mg daily and increase gradually to 5000mg daily (not with meals) for most symptoms

Phospholipids, including lecithin, are important in the transmission of nerve impulses. Lecithin also helps promote the secretion of glandular hormones and mental alertness.

DOSAGE:

Lecithin	1 tablespoon with food 3 times daily

Ringworm

This affliction has nothing to do with worms. It is actually a fungus infection of the skin, hair or nails. The infection causes inflammation of the skin and the raised outer edge of the ring looks like a worm. The inflamed skin becomes spongy and flakes and peels, causing intense itchiness. School children are particularly prone to ringworm of the body which they catch when in contact with infected children. It can also be contracted from animals, in particular cats.

Treatment requires the skin to be kept dry so the fungus cannot grow. Care must be taken to avoid contact with contaminated sheets, towels and clothing. If the affliction has spread through the family then all linen must be sterilised or boiled. Anti-fungal creams can be used or tea tree oil applied to the area is very effective.

Ringworm of the scalp is common amongst boys who catch it from seats, at the barber shop, or swapping hats. Tea tree shampoo will help kill the fungus. It is wise to start treating it as soon as it is diagnosed as the condition may cause hair loss, splitting of the hair and scaliness.

Shock

Shock is a sharp fall in blood pressure and the consequent drop in the blood reaching tissues and the brain. The causes include loss of body fluid to blood loss, a heart attack or decreased blood pressure as a result of a spinal injury or poisoning. Rapid treatment is critical as the condition may lead to the collapse of the circulatory system and death.

The symptoms are a pale face and clammy skin, a weak pulse and fast breathing, a feeling of being faint, and nausea. In cases of severe shock the extremities of the body may turn blue and the patient becomes thirsty. To treat shock, lay the patient down, loosen tight clothing, keep the person warm but not hot, do not give them anything to eat or drink (although you can moisten their lips), make sure they can breathe and keep a record of the pulse. If there is difficulty breathing, the patient is losing consciousness or there is a chance of vomiting, lay the patient on their side.

If breathing stops start Expired Air Resuscitation (mouth-to-mouth breathing). If the patient is unconscious and no pulse is detected start CPR (cardio pulmonary resuscitation) immediately and seek medical aid.

Sinusitis

This painful condition may cause a lot of disruption in childhood and adolescence, with school absence and pain. It is so hard to concentrate when afflicted. The cause is an inflammation of the mucous membranes which line the air-filled cavities or sinuses in the bones of the face and skull. The symptoms are headache, toothache-like pain, aching eyes and loss of sense of smell.

It is advisable for the sufferer to avoid dairy products as these can be mucous-forming. The herbs horseradish and garlic can help dry out the sinuses and can be taken in tablet form. Garlic is very helpful as it is Nature's antibiotic and can reduce the infection which causes inflammation of the area. Vitamin A will help to strengthen the mucous membranes in the nose and throat, and the essential fatty acids that are a part of cod liver oil help relieve inflammation and pain. As both vitamin A and the omega-3 essential fatty acids can be found in cod liver oil, supplementation may help.

SUPPLEMENTS

cod liver oil	over 6 years take 5mls (1 tspn) just before food daily (to strengthen mucous membranes)
horseradish /garlic	1 tablet just after food up to 3 times daily
vitamin C	6 to 12 years take 250mg daily 12 years and over and adults take up to 2,000mg daily

NASAL SPRAY FORMULA
Use when required to relieve congestion.

salt	1 tspn
glycerin	1 tspn
eucalyptus oil	1 drop
boiled water	600ml

Use the above formula to fill a nasal spray bottle and squirt up both nostrils to flush out congestion.

Snoring

If you or a member of your family snore then it could be the result of nasal congestion or sinus problems (see also SINUSITIS). It also could be caused by enlarged adenoids. Usually snoring is caused by the soft palate at the back of the mouth vibrating, resulting in the snoring sound.

Snoring is not usually anything to worry about. However, noisy breathing and snoring can accompany a head injury or overdose of sleeping tablets or alcohol. If your child normally does not sore and does not have a cold then check that medication has not been taken accidentally. Sometimes a little shake to disturb the sleep will stop the snoring.

SUPPLEMENTS
Same as for Sinusitis

Sore throat and tonsillitis

Every person will get a sore throat at some time in their life. Minor viral infections are common in school years. A diet high in fresh fruit and vegetables will help build resistance to infections. Tonsillitis is another common cause of a painful and infected throat in young children usually between the ages of 2 to 8 years. If the child has a fever, finds it difficult to swallow and the throat is painful, then check the tonsils to see if they are enlarged and red. They also usually will have pus blotches on them. This can easily be seen as yellow and white patches on the tonsils situated at either side of the back of the throat.

Gargling with warm salty water is helpful as it kills bacteria and reduces the swelling. The herbs echinacea and garlic can be very helpful in combating sore throats and tonsillitis. These herbs have anti-microbial properties and can stimulate the immune system. Vitamin C can be helpful. If your child isn't eating enough fresh fruit and vegetables which contain vitamin C, supplementation will reduce symptoms. Cod liver oil can be helpful in the treatment of sore throats and infections. It can help reduce inflammation and strengthen the mucous lining of the throat.

Infections that don't respond to treatment or continually occur should be discussed with your practitioner. Although surgical removal is usually not indicated, in severe cases antibiotics may be needed.

SUPPLEMENTS

cod liver oil	1 to 6 years 2.5ml
	just before food once daily
	6 years and over 5ml before food daily
echinacea	children 6 to 12 years take
	1/2 tablet with food twice daily
	adults 1 tablet daily
vitamin C	children 2 to 6 years crush
	child's chewable vitamin C
	with food once daily
	6 to 12 years 250mg daily
	12 years and over 1,000mg daily

Stress and vitamin B

Most vitamin B complexes are formulated for different complaints; there are stress formulas, PMT formulas and general vitamin B formulas to compensate for dietary vitamin B deficiencies. Let us first examine what the B complex vitamins are and what they do.

All the B vitamins are water soluble and the single B vitamins that make up a vitamin B complex are: vitamin B1 (thiamin), vitamin B2 (riboflavin), vitamin B3 (niacin), vitamin B5 (pantothenic acid), vitamin B6 (pyridoxine), vitamin B12 (cyanocobalamin), biotin and folic acid. Other important nutrients that are included as part of the vitamin B complex, although not true vitamins, are PABA, choline and inositol.

These vitamins and nutrients can be cultivated from bacteria, fungi, moulds or brewer's yeast. Brewer's yeast is one of the best sources as it contains all the B vitamins with the exception of vitamin B17.

The B complex of vitamins is required by our bodies to convert carbohydrates into glucose. This conversion gives us the energy required for day-to-day activity. These important nutrients are also essential for healthy skin, eyes, mouth, liver, muscle tone and a healthy nervous system.

Vitamin B complex has been used and proven in clinical studies to be beneficial when used for the treatment of some nervous disorders including anxiety, depression and premenstrual tension.

For us to keep up with the pace of modern-day life in this stressful and fast moving world we need to ensure that our diets include wholegrain cereals, brewer's yeast, dairy products, and meat. These foods are good sources of all the B vitamins; however, even if we are eating correctly the absorption and/or utilisation of B vitamins can be adversely affected by our lifestyle and medications.

The contraceptive pill, sleeping tablets, sulpha drugs, and certain antibiotics can cause an imbalance in the digestive tract that can destroy B vitamins at a fast rate as can stress and infection. For these reasons, if you suffer from stress or illness, or you are taking any of the aforementioned medications, I recommend that you supplement your diet with a B complex. This will give nutritional insurance against vitamin B deficiency. But still the question arises, which complex should you choose?

Look for a supplement that contains the minerals potassium phosphate and magnesium phosphate. These two cell salts have been used for decades in the clinical management of certain types of stress. Webb et al reported in *Psychosomatics* 22(3),199-203, 1981, that low blood potassium is frequently associated with tearfulness, weakness, and fatigue. It was also found that even though blood levels of potassium were normal, intracellular potassium was low in patients suffering from depression. Low magnesium has also been found to be associated with depression.

To make a vitamin B stress formula even more complete, the addition of vitamin C and stress-relieving herbs is a must. Vitamin C, found in fresh fruit and vegetables, is also needed by your body to help you cope with stress.

The herbs that should be included are valerian, passion flower and scullcap. These herbs have been used for centuries for the treatment of stress and anxiety and are mentioned in the *British Herbal Pharmacopoeia* as calming herbs.

In summary, if you suffer from stress and you would like some help in coping, then, take time out to relax, exercise a little each day, eat well and consider supplementing your diet with a B stress formula containing the nutrients and herbs that I have mentioned.

Sty

Infection can cause a small abscess in the gland of the eyelid. It appears as a red swelling and may form a head with pus in it. This may break naturally.

A warm compress will bring relief as the pain is acute. Put half a teaspoon of salt in a medium sized bowl of warm water. Soak and squeeze a folded triangle of clean cloth and apply to the eye for 20 minutes every hour and a half. This will help the sty come to a head and will also relieve the pain. In some children the sty will recur frequently and cause continued discomfort.

Bathe the eye and the eye area with an eye wash formula made from the herb golden seal. Supplementing with the herb echinacea can help build the immune system and minimise recurrence of the sty.

SUPPLEMENTS

echinacea	liquid extract or dried herb in tablet form as directed on bottle
vitamin C	children over 6 years 250 mg daily 12 years and over take 1,000mg tablet morning and night

(For eye bath formula see CONJUNCTIVITIS)

Sunburn

Infants and young children are easily burnt (see also BURNS) by the ultraviolet rays from the sun and it is now thought that early exposure to the sun can dramatically increase the danger of skin cancer in later life. Hats and sunscreens must be part of the process of going to the beach and in some schools it is now compulsory for children to wear hats in the playground. Covering the legs on the beach is also important as the sun's rays are reflected off the sand.

When sunburn has occurred the person must be given plenty of fluids to stop dehydration and cool compresses need to be applied to the burnt skin. An aloe vera cream or better still the juice of the aloe vera plant will help prevent moisture loss and promote healing - it is one of the best treatments for burns. As the child begins to recover from the burn, to help the growth of new skin, use a vitamin E cream and supplement with vitamins E, C and the mineral zinc.

If an infant or child develops blisters after sunburning it is necessary to seek advice from your practitioner.

SUPPLEMENTS

Children's Chewable Multi Vitamin	2 to 6 years of age 1 tablet daily 6 to 12 years 500mg vitamin C
zinc	12 years and over take 1 tablet daily with food

vitamin C 1,000mg   take 1 tablet with food morning
                       and night

Thrush (see Candidiasis)

Tinea (see Ringworms, Nappyrash)

Warts

Sometimes adolescents will have an outbreak of warts on
the hands or feet. They are a viral skin infection and picking at
them will only make the problem worse. They are best treated
with an ointment, the most effective being thuja. This herb can
be applied externally twice daily to the wart which should be kept
covered. Keep up the treatment until the wart drops off. Building
up the immune system to help defeat the virus is also helpful. The
herb echinacea, vitamins A, C and E, zinc and garlic will all help
to prevent a recurrence of the warts.

SUPPLEMENTS

	adult dosage
echinacea	500mg 3 times daily
vitamin A	10,000iu daily
vitamin C	4,000mg daily
vitamin E	500iu daily
garlic	equivalent of 2,000mg fresh herb daily

ointment containing thuja applied 3 times daily

Weight loss and hot foods

You may feel that when you eat hot food such as chilli,
mustard or peppers that they are not good for you. These foods
indeed can and do give a burning sensation to the mucous
membranes in your mouth and because these foods are so 'HOT'
many of us just can't eat them.

Hot foods they may be but chillies can help you lose

weight! Yes, the latest studies using chilli, mustard seeds and spices showed that weight loss can be increased by as much as 25 per cent when these spices are added to a calorie controlled diet. Chillies, or cayenne pepper, as they are more commonly known, have been used as a remedy for intestinal wind and poor digestion for hundreds of years and today they are still included in many people's diet in order to obtain these benefits.

Scientists now believe that two of the chemicals found in cayenne could increase weight loss by their action upon the thyroid hormone. A study carried out at the University of Tasmania found that the metabolic rate of 4 out of 6 people was increased after one meal which contained one tablespoon of tabasco.

If being overweight is your problem, then add a little of the 'HOT STUFF' to your meals either by sprinkling it on or adding it when cooking. Cayenne pepper can be bought from your health food store in bulk and it is not expensive; however it is hot, so only use a little at first and build up to about a quarter of a teaspoon at each meal. This should do the trick.

If you can't stand the heat, then take an empty capsule and fill it with 300mg of cayenne pepper. You should then take one with each meal. Sometimes hot spicy foods can upset the stomach and if this is the case then reduce the amount or discontinue their use.

Remember, if you are serious about weight loss then don't eat junk foods. Chocolate, sausage rolls and milk shakes as part of the daily diet will still put on weight even if you do add chilli. Eat lots of vegetables and fruit, and include whole grains, lean meat and low fat dairy products in your diet. This, in conjunction with chillies, will not only help you maintain your correct weight but keep you a lot more healthy.

Drink more water to help the body to be flushed of toxins. Also water is a food appetite suppressant. Six to eight glasses per day are needed for good health.

Exercise is also very important as during exercise the metabolic rate increases and you will burn up kilojoules more quickly, resulting in a reduction in weight and a healthier you.

PART III

Guide to herbs in this book

ALFALFA (Lucerne)
Medicago sativa
Description: A perennial herb from 30 to 80 cms in height, trifoliate leaves, blue to purple flowers in summer which vary in size and colour depending on cultivation.

Uses: The leaves contain beta-carotene, vitamins C, D, E, and K; and mineral salts, calcium, potassium, iron and phosphorus, making the plant nutritious. The leaves can be steamed or eaten raw in salads or soups. Tea is said to be good for digestion, appetite increase, and as a multi vitamin and mineral source.

ALOE
Aloe vera, Aloe barbandensis, Aloe perryi and *Aloe ferrox*
Description: Aloe vera is one of the 200 succulents from the genus Aloe, and lily family. Leaves grow from the central stem and produce a juice. The flowers are red.

Uses: The juice from Cape aloes can act as a purgative. For gastric disorders, colitis, peptic ulcers and externally (for burns, bites, bruises, and as a cosmetic for skin and hair) it is used.

ANISEED
Pimpinella anisum
Description: Aromatic annual, native to Turkey and Greece, up to 60 cm, upper leaves pinnate, yellow flowers in umbels in summer which produce fruit.

Uses: The seed aids digestion and can be cooked or made into tea which alleviates flatulence, cramps, nausea, diarrhoea, colic, hiccups, insomnia, and chest complaints.

BARBERRY
Berberis vulgaris
Description: A deciduous shrub to 3m, with spines on the branches, oval leaves, yellow flowers in summer, and red oblong berries.

Uses:The bark of the plant affects the liver and the gall bladder (particularly gallstones) and is used in cases of jaundice and gastric problems. It can be used to treat nausea and as a mouthwash is effective for sore throats. It should be avoided in early pregnancy.

BAYBERRY
Myrica cerifera
Description: Bayberry varies from a small evergreen shrub to a tree that can reach a height of 10m. The fruit looks like a small cluster of wax covered berries.

Uses: Commonly used to treat diarrhoea and mucous colitis. Bayberry is also used as a gargle for sore throats and colds.

BEARBERRY
(see Uva ursi)

BETONY
Betonica officinalis
Description: A perennial to 60 cm, squarish stems, hairy leaves at the base, and a dense spike of pink to purple flowers in summer to autumn.

Uses: A tincture made from the above-ground parts is used for diarrhoea. It has mild sedative properties and can aid in the relief of headaches and anxiety. It has also been used in treatment of rheumatism, varicose veins, and is said to be a tonic for children who are not growing normally. Beware of using the root as it may cause vomiting.

BLACK COHOSH
Cimicifuga racemosa
Description: A tall, feathery, herbaceous plant up to 3

metres with dry white flowers which droop. The rhizome is black and knotty where the dried ascending stems once were. The fresh root is used to make a tincture.

Uses: This herb can be used in the acute stage of rheumatoid arthritis and sciatica. It also relieves menstrual cramps and stimulates contractions of the uterus in childbirth. It is an effective stimulant for the heart and lowers high blood pressure, is a sedative for the nervous system and can also be used in cases of hysteria. It can also be used in combination with *Ginkgo biloba* for tinnitus or ringing in the ears.

BLUEBERRY (Bilberry)
Vaccinium myrtillus
Description :   A low shrub to 50 cm with oval leaves, greenish-pink flowers in spring, and blue-black berries.

Uses: The leaves contain glucoquinine which lowers blood sugar level. The berries, which contain vitamin C, can be dried and used for circulatory problems, the treatment of diabetes, burns, ulcers, inflamed gums, and catarrh. They also help improve night vision and circulation to the eyes. This herb could be useful in adjunctive treatment of many ophthalmic conditions.

BOLDO
Peumus boldus
Description: An aromatic bush with opposite leaves which originates in Chile and produces compounds that are cholagogic.

Uses: Stimulates the secretion of bile, the liver, the gall bladder, the digestive acids, the pancreas, and acts as a diuretic. Specific uses are as a liver tonic and for treatment of painful gallstones.

BUCKTHORN
Rhamnus catharticus
Description: A deciduous shrub to 5m with spreading branches, very small greenish flowers with 4 petals, male and female on separate plants, and black fleshy fruits.

Uses: The bark of this plant can be used as a powerful

diuretic and purgative which is used in cases of chronic constipation. Do not use the fresh bark as it is too strong. The fruits are a diuretic and a purgative.

BURDOCK
Arctium lappa

Description: A weed native to North America and Europe which produces burrs after flowering. The root, large leaves and the seeds are used.

Uses: Burdock is used for liver, skin and kidney problems, the stomach and the blood. Externally it is applied to bruises, sprains, acne, eczema and boils.

CAMPHOR LAUREL
Cinnamomum camphora

Description: A large tree to 50m which can live for 1,000 years. The leaves are aromatic and insect-repelling storage chests are carved from the strong smelling timber.

Uses: The oil is contained in the leaves and branches and is commonly used on inflamed joints but is also used in small doses as a sedative. It was used as an antispasmodic for epilepsy. Internally, fresh camphor can stimulate the heart and lungs. Applied externally it relieves sprains and strains. Large doses are toxic to children.

CASCARA SAGRADA
Rhamnus purshiana

Description: A many branched shrub to 2 metres, native to North Africa. The main stem is black, branches ash colour terminating in a thorn. Leaves grow in bunches and fruit is pea-size and black with 4 brown seeds.

Uses: *Cascara sagrada* affects the liver, gallbladder, colon, stomach and pancreas. It is a laxative, anti-spasmodic and hepatic tonic. It can be used in either the tincture or dried herb form. Cascara is used whenever haemorrhoids are associated with constipation and poor bowel function. It is also very useful for bowel-related problems in combination with bayberry bark, rhubarb root, golden seal and raspberry leaves as a lower bowel tonic. The flesh of birds that eat this herb is said to be purgative.

CASSIA
Cassia senna
Description: There are many species of trees and shrubs in the genus Cassia, characterised by bright yellow flowers and pods containing many seeds. The species determines which part of the plant is used, ranging from leaves, seeds, pods, to the bark.
Uses: Depending on the species and the part of the plant used, cassia can treat constipation and is a cathartic medicine. The dried pods and leaves are used as a strong laxative.

CAYENNE
Capsicum minimum
Description: There are over 50 cultivated peppers, an annual with a green, red or orange elongated fruit in late spring.
Uses: The dried, ground powder taken internally can improve circulation, digestion and relieve flatulence. A weak solution can be used for a throat gargle. Used externally paprika can soothe rheumatism, arthritis, chilblains and pleurisy.

CELERY
Apium graveolens
Description: A biennial which grows to the height of 1m and has a characteristic smell. The vegetable is recommended as a diuretic and appetite suppressant.
Uses: The seeds are used for treating rheumatism and anxiety. Celery seeds are of great value in the treatment of arthritis and gout.

CHICKWEED
Stellaria media
Description: Related to groundsel, the stems are long and leggy, tailing on the ground. Leaves are succulent and pale green, opposite, and smooth. The flowers are white, single, and small. At night the leaves enfold the new shoots.

Uses: Rich in nutrients and vitamins A, B, and C, it eases constipation and inflammation of the digestive system. Externally it can be applied to haemorrhoids, skin irritations, eczema, chilblains, carbuncles and abcesses.

CLOVES
Eugenia caryophyllata
Description: A small tree, divided trunk with many branches, smooth, bright green, aromatic leaves. The flowers are pale orange fading to yellow, then red. The cloves are contained in the calyx and are beaten from the tree before they age and lose their aroma.
Uses: The oil is used for toothache, and also for flatulence, dyspepsia, nausea and colic. It should be stored in a dark bottle in a cool place.

COMFREY
Symphytum officinale
Description: A member of the borage group, the plant is a clump of hairy leaves with a deep root which draws nutrients from the soil. The lower leaves can be up to 20 cms long, decreasing in size as they go up the stem.
Uses: The foliage and root of this plant contain a nitrogenous, crystalline substance called allantoin which is a cell proliferant. It has a soothing and healing effect upon every organ it comes in contact with. Comfrey may be taken internally or used externally for broken bones, sores and because of the cell-growing action, speeds up healing. A poultice of freshly bruised leaves applied to a burn or wound, will increase the healing process and minimise inflammation. In Ireland the fresh young leaves are eaten to improve the blood and circulation. NOTE, Comfrey is poisonous and in large amounts, or for long periods of time, is cumulative. Seek advice from your naturopath.

CORN SILK
Zea mays
Description: The stigmas or long fine hairs on the female

fruit are the silk. The fruit in autumn has yellow, red, purple or brown kernel on a cob.

Uses: Combined with agrimony and made into a tea it is used to treat bedwetting. Also used as a diuretic, for prostate problems, bladder irritations, and in the treatment of prostatitis.

COUCH GRASS
Agropyrum repens
Description: A grass with a slender rhizome, hollow stems up to half a metre high, with 5 to 7 leaves. The leaves are flat and rough on top with a central vein.

Uses: Possessing antibiotic qualities, it acts as an antiseptic diuretic and is used commonly with bladder complaints and prostatic enlargements when combined with hydrangea.

CRANESBILL
Geranium maculatum
Description: A perennial up to half a metre in height, it is erect, hairy and branchless. The leaves are cleft and toothed and the flowers are rosy pink. The fruit has five cells each containing seeds. The root is brown, white inside, 4 to 8 cms and covered in branchlets. This is the part used.

Uses: In cases of diarrhoea, haemorrhoids, peptic ulcers, thrush, and haemorrhaging in the digestive tract. It can be used as a mouthwash for mouth ulcers and sore throats as a gargle.

DANDELION
Taraxacum officinale
Description: Leaves grow in a rosette on the ground from which emerges a central stalk with milky sap. The flower is yellow and has a pungent smell. The root is a thick brown tap root. The name comes from the French for lion's tooth, *dent de lion*. Leaves and the root are used.

Uses: Dandelion affects the kidneys, gallbladder, liver, pancreas and blood. Its main use would be for liver complaints or as a diuretic. Dandelion stimulates the liver increasing its detoxifying action. Because of this action dandelion is a valuable blood purifying herb and may be used in some skin diseases. Dandelion is also a very useful diuretic. The dandelion leaves can be eaten as part of a salad and will help prevent liver problems and gallstones. The dried roots are roasted and used to make a coffee substitute. It is a tonic for dyspepsia and a laxative in mild constipation.

DILL
Anethum graveolens

Description: An annual with one stalk up to three-quarters of a metre, with feathery leaves and flowers in an umbrella shape (like fennel) which are yellow. Small black seeds are produced in autumn.

Uses: Fresh as a flavouring with potatoes, eggs, chicken, and fish, it is a popular summer culinary herb. The seeds can be made into a tea to ease indigestion and children's colic.

DONG QUAI
Angelica sinensis

Description: Long thin roots, bold metre long reddish purple foliage to 2m, greenish-white flowers in the umbel or umbrella like formation of dill and fennel. The plant is extremely fragrant in all parts. The rhizome is used.

Uses: Dong quai is used in the treatment of most female gynaecological ailments, in particular menstrual cramps, premenstrual tension, menopause and irregularity. It is used to treat hot flushes during menopause and is also nourishing to the blood, being rich in vitamin E and vitamin B12. It is also useful in the treatment of anaemia. Dong quai is very useful in combination with other herbs such as black cohosh, queen of the meadow, red raspberry, blessed thistle, and *Vitex agnus-castus*.

ECHINACEA (Purple coneflower)
Echinacea angustifolia

Description: The plant has purple flowers, a tapering root, thin bark, an aromatic smell and sweet taste.

Uses: This herb is used both internally and externally, to increase the body's resistance to infection, for boils, acne, abscesses, severe bites, septicaemia, fevers, and in some cases it has been used to treat cancer. It is a dilator of peripheral blood vessels. It is mentioned in the *British Herbal Pharmacopaeia* as an anti-viral herb, truly a herb of the future.

ELDER FLOWER
Sambucus nigra

Description: A familiar tree in England, it bears creamy white flowers in terminals that are followed by large purplish-black bunches of berries. The flowers, berries, leaves and bark have different properties and are used in many ways.

Uses: The flowers of the black elder are used as an ingredient in eye lotion and for skin complaints. They are mainly used to treat colds, sinus, chronic nasal catarrh with deafness, throat infections, and in combination with other herbs, constipation, diarrhoea, bronchitis, cystitis, and fluid retention. The leaves are dried and used in ointments for sprains, bruises and cuts. Like the leaves, the bark is a purgative. Leaves can also be used for eye infections. The berries are made into wine in Europe. It is mainly used for sinusitis and the common cold.

EPHEDRA
Ephedra vulgaris

Description: A plant growing in temperate climates, unusual for the stamens and pistils appearing on separate flowers and fruit which is a succulent cone.

Uses: It is a potent stimulant of the nervous system and is used for bronchial asthma, hayfever, skin complaints, purifying the blood, and low blood pressure. Many modern medicines are based on this herb.

EUCALYPTUS
Eucalyptus globulus

Description: Native to Tasmania, the blue gum has large leathery leaves studded with oil glands which are highly aromatic. The flowers appear in large creamy clusters. It is one of the tallest species of eucalypt.

Uses: The oil is used as an aromatic and antiseptic. Externally it is used for burns, cuts, ulcers, and sores. Inhaled, it clears the nose and lungs, relieves the symptoms of bronchitis and asthma. It can also be used as an insect repellant.

EUPHORBIA
Euphorbia hirta

Description: A leafless perennial up to a metre in height which resembles a cactus. It has small, bright yellow flowers.

Uses: Relaxes the bronchi and is used to treat asthma. The latex is used to treat warts. Its main uses are as an anti-asthmatic and for upper respiratory catarrh.

EVENING PRIMROSE
Oenothera biennis

Description: Named evening primrose because the flowers usually open in the evening, it is a biennial plant. In the first year flattened leaves grow at ground level. In the second year a stem grows from the centre to over 1m. It produces fragrant yellow flowers in summer.

Uses: The oil extracted from the seeds contains omega-6 fatty acids such as GLA. The oil is used for coughs, colds, gastrointestinal and menstrual problems and for menopausal depression. The oil is used internally and externally for skin eruptions and sores. Primrose oil can also help lower cholesterol and blood pressure. Many clinical studies and trials have been done using Efamol, a brand of evening primrose oil, with very positive results in the treatment of eczema and other skin disorders.

EYEBRIGHT
Euphrasia officinalis

Description: A small annual which grows on limestone based soils. The leaves are deeply cut and the flowers are white to purple with yellow markings.

Uses: Used in eye lotion for conjunctivitis, it possesses anti-inflammatory qualities for ailments of the eyes. Main uses are upper respiratory catarrh, sinusitis and conjuctivitis.

FENNEL
Foeniculum vulgare
Description: It has the typical feathery foliage and umbrella formation of the flowers of the umbelliferous herbs, closely resembling the dill plant. It is hardy and grows along roadsides throughout Australia, flowering in summer.

Uses: A tea made from the seeds relieves flatulence, stimulates the pancreas, and is recommended for weight loss, nursing mothers, and diabetes. Mixed with dill and peppermint, it treats flatulence in infants.

FENUGREEK
Trigonella foenum-graecum
Description: This erect herb grows to well over a metre and produces bitter angular seeds, brown and divided into two lobes.

Uses: It is a popular culinary herb in Indian cooking. Aids in bronchitis, catarrh, sinus, digestion of fatty foods and acne. A paste can be applied to boils and wounds.

FEVERFEW
Chrysanthemum parthenium
Description: Feverfew is a member of the chrysanthemum family and grows as a weed in many gardens. It has many daisy-like flowers, yellow and white and the yellow centre is flat. It is a perennial and has a strong smell which repels bees.

Uses: It is used as a tonic for nervousness, promotes menstruation, prevents migraine, headache, fever, tension. It repels insects, it is said to be good to plant around the house.

GARLIC
Allium sativum
Description: Belonging to the onion family, garlic has long flat leaves above the ground and a large bulb, made up of many

smaller bulbs, underground.

Uses: Garlic is a natural antimicrobial and helps protect us against the common cold, infectious diseases such as typhoid and dysentery and lung disorders. It increases flow of bile from liver, can be used to treat bronchitis, as well as some intestinal ailments such as candida. It is also used in treatment of high blood pressure and hardening of the arteries.

GENTIAN
Gentiana lutea
Description: A hardy herbaceous perennial with yellow-orange flowers. The root is long and thick (25 cm), the stem is over a metre long with leaves opposite at all joints. Strong plants produce abundant seeds.

Uses: The bitter vegetable tonic is used to treat exhaustion, appetite and digestion, in such cases as debility and anorexia.

GINGER
Zingiber officinale
Description: Grows from a rhizome underground which sends up green shoots in spring and a fragrant flower in summer. The root is the part of the plant used and it is dried and powdered or the oil is extracted.

Uses: Used for stomach disorders where there is no inflammation, motion sickness, menstruation pain, improving circulation and alcoholic gastritis.

GINSENG
Panax ginseng
Description: A perennial herb which is native to China, Manchuria and Korea. It has a fleshy ringed root that forks into two at the end and is usually gold or brown. The stem is simple and grows to 60 to 80 cm, bears three to five palmate leaves, yellow flowers and bright red berries.

Uses: In China ginseng was so highly valued that for thousands of years wars were fought for the possession of this herb. It is used to increase mental and physical efficiency and can reduce blood pressure and cholesterol and suppress development of cancer cells, bolstering the immune system. Its action on the endocrine glands should increase vitamin and mineral utilisation. It has also been used to treat masculine sexual potency.

GLOBE ARTICHOKE
Cynara scolymus
Description: A member of the same family as the Scottish thistle, it looks something like a giant thistle, particularly when it flowers, producing a saucer-sized purple spiky bloom. The mature vegetable stands on a stem 1 to 1.5 metres with the purple green artichoke on top.

Uses: Usually eaten as a delicacy, this vegetable treats jaundice and liver insufficiency. As a heart stimulant, it is a prophylactic against arteriosclerosis and helps lower cholesterol.

GOLDEN SEAL
Hydrastis canadensis
Description: A native to Canada, golden seal is from the same family as buttercups. It grows on a single stem, has two leaves with several lobes and a spring flower which has three sepals, no petals and many stamens. It produces a red berry. The root is used.

Uses: It can be taken for stomach and menstrual disorders. It causes oversecretion of mucous membranes, especially the uterus and relieves sinusitis and catarrh. It is a powerful antiseptic and antimicrobial which can be used for many diseases of the gastro-intestinal tract. It is used as a very effective eye wash and treats any inflammation of the eyes.

GRINDELIA
Grindelia camporum
Description: A biennial, perennial or small shrub with round yellow stems, smooth alternate leaves at the base, and

bristles around the flower heads. It is native to North and South America. The leaves and flower heads are used.

Uses: Works as an expectorant and mild sedative for relief of respiratory tract infections and asthma. Also to treat catarrh of the urinary tract and bladder.

GUAIACUM
Guaiacum officinale
Description: An evergreen tree with purplish-blue flowers, from the West Indies, which grows to 20 metres. A resin is extracted from the bark and timber.

Uses: To relieve the pain of rheumatism, gout and arthritis, it also works as an antiseptic and diuretic.

HAWTHORN
Crataegus monogyna
Description: A small deciduous tree which grows in cold climates in Australia, for example New England and the ACT. It has small white flowers in spring and red berries in autumn and is covered in thorns. The dried fruit is used.

Uses: It is specifically used to treat the muscular action of the heart in conditions such as irregular heartbeat, palpitations, angina, arteriosclerosis, circulatory disorders, and blood pressure.

HOPS
Humulus lupulus
Description: Native to Britain, hops are related to stinging nettles, have a twining stem which is prickly, and heart-shaped leaves which are opposite. Male and female flowers are on separate plants and the female produces the fruit, or cone, that is used commercially. In a plantation of hops, such as Tasmania, only a few males will be found, for fertilisation purposes.

Uses: As a soporific to treat insomnia, anxiety, indigestion, and also for the relief of menstrual pain and neuralgia. It is drunk as a tea in Britain to induce sleep and calm the nerves.

HOREHOUND

Marrubium vulgare

Description: Native to Britain, it is a bushy annual to 25cms with woolly white flowers in whorls.

Uses: Beneficial for disorders of the gall bladder and the stomach, it can also be used to treat menstrual pain. It is specifically of use in bronchial disorders for congestion and the loosening of phlegm. It is drunk as a tea made from the leaves.

HORSERADISH
Cochlearia amoracia

Description: Native to Europe, horseradish grows like a radish with long green leaves and a fleshy white root with enlarged crown being produced in summer.

Uses: Eaten raw, it stimulates digestion. It clears the head and relieves congestion of the sinuses. It works as a diuretic and fresh root scraped can be applied externally for rheumatism and neuralgia. It is mainly used in combination with garlic for sinusitis.

HORSETAIL
Equisetum arvense

Description: Horsetail is native to Britain. It has threadlike foliage that is jointed, grows from a rhizome and is similar to ferns in that it produces spores. The slender fronds have a high silica content and were once used in Europe to clean metal.

Uses: A potent diuretic, it can be drunk as a tea to remove gall or kidney stones and can assist in prostate problems. It promotes coagulation and corpuscle growth, reducing internal and external bleeding.

IRISH MOSS
Chondrus crispus

Description: Known as 'carrageen', it occurs at low tide on the shores of the North Atlantic. Irish moss is a gum derived from seaweed and is used in pharmaceutical products.

Uses: Its soothing properties are useful for bronchial and digestive irritations, treatment of the heart, bladder and kidneys.

Irish moss is high in mucilage and iodine and its main use is for coughs and colds.

JUNIPER
Juniperus communis
Description: Common in Europe, the commercial berries are grown in Hungary. It is a shrub to over 1 metre in height producing blue berries after three years.

Uses: It is used commercially in the production of gin. It is effective used internally as a urinary antiseptic and to stimulate appetite. The oil can be used in a vaporiser for bronchial infections. The berries are said to prevent water retention. Juniper should not be used during pregnancy.

KELP
Fucus vesiculosis
Description: This kelp's frond is coarse and yellow, growing on rocks exposed at low tide. It grows to a metre in length, is fan shaped, leathery and has smooth edges. It is harvested in summer and dried immediately in the sun.

Uses: Kelp is high in iodine, beta-carotene and minerals and used in the treatment of disorders of the thyroid gland and to treat obesity when associated with hypothyroidism.

KOLA
Cola nitida
Description: Kola grows in equatorial regions. It is a tree up to 12 metres in height which has yellow flowers followed by seeds.

Uses: It contains caffeine and is a heart stimulant. It is used to treat headaches, migraine and depression.

LIME FLOWERS
Tilia cordata
Description: A British tree that grows to 35 metres, has heart shaped leaves and long clusters of flowers, used for honey

production and tea making. It is called the linden tree.

Uses: In combination with hawthorn and mistletoe, the flowers can be used to treat hypertension. The flowers of the lime are used for palpitations, nervousness and indigestion.

LIQUORICE
Glycyrrhiza glabra
Description: The plant has graceful foliage which hangs down at night. It produces lilac flowers which are followed by a smooth pod. It has a long taproot with many spreading roots which send up shoots. Native to the Mediterranean and Asia, it is a nitrogen fixing plant.

Uses: Liquorice treats respiratory complaints and is known for its laxative properties. It is also used as an anti-inflammatory medicine, possessing similar qualities to prednizone. Pregnant women, diabetics, and anyone suffering hypertension or kidney complaints should check with their practitioners before taking liquorice in large amounts. Liquorice was an effective treatment for Addison's disease as liquorice causes sodium retention. Addison's disease causes sodium excretion.

MILK THISTLE
Silybum marianum
Description: A weed in Britain, it was once a cultivated garden plant, tall with glossy leaves marked by white veins. All parts of the plant are used.

Uses: The milk thistle leaves are thought to help produce milk in nursing mothers, the powdered seeds can also be used in certain cardiovascular disorders. The root and seeds stimulate the liver and spleen and the actives in this herb protect the liver from toxins including alcohol, and are helpful in the treatment of hepatitis and other liver diseases.

MULLEIN
Verbascum thapsus
Description: Mullein is in the same family as the snapdrag-

ons but flowers are unspectacular. Leaves resemble comfrey and the flowers appear on a 1 to 2 metre rod and are stalkless and chrome-yellow. It is a hairy plant. Leaves, flowers and roots are used.

Uses: Specifically used for respiratory disorders, working as an expectorant and a sedative. Externally an oil from the flowers can treat haemorrhoids, bruises, nappy rash and warts. Generally, for treating inflammation of the mucous membranes.

OATS
Avena sativa
Description: A cereal which grows annually and resembles wheat with a smooth stem to over one metre, but differs in that the grains fall naked from the husk.

Uses: Oats are nutritious and soothe the intestinal tract, are good for the heart and relieve nervous anxiety. The meal is used externally for skin disorders and the dried straw is used as tea for chest complaints. Oats are particularly useful in the treatment of menopausal depression and other mild depressive states.

OLIVE OIL
Olea europaea
Description: The European olive is a small tree with dark green leaves above and silvery below. The flowers are creamy white and the fruit is a purple drupe which contains oil. They grow well in Australia, particularly around Perth and Adelaide.

Uses: Olive oil can be absorbed by babies through the skin and in adults the oil is used on bruises, burns and bites, and softens dry skin and hair. It is useful for muscular, chest, kidney and abdominal complaints and disperses acids and toxins in the blood. It is thought to lower cholesterol and is nutritious for people of all ages.

OREGANO
Origanum vulgare
Description: A perennial herb grown for culinary purposes, with creeping roots, woody stems and small leaves. Its flowers

are rose-purple to pink on a short spike and the whole plant smells like balsam.

Uses: Used mainly as an expectorant and antispasmodic in cough formulas. Oregano is also an antiseptic and is used in a tea for nervous headache.

PASSION FLOWER
Passiflora incarnata
Description: One of the many members of the Passifloraceae family. The common passion fruit (P. edulis) is well-known in the backyard, with its three lobed leaf and purple fruit.

Uses: In the treatment of insomnia, nervousness and anxiety, it is also employed to treat types of convulsion and also epilepsy. It depresses the motor nerves.

PEPPERMINT
Mentha piperita
Description: Long purple stems, leaves have toothed margins, smooth surfaces and a distinctive vein on the underside. The flowers are in whorls and are reddish purple in colour.

Uses: The oil has anti-spasmodic qualities and is used to treat gastro intestinal disorders, internal circulation, agitation and headaches. It is a good cordial for infants with colic.

PLEURISY ROOT
Asclepias tuberosa
Description: A perennial growing in peat soils, the root is used. It produces orange to yellow flowers in autumn.

Uses: Specifically for the use of respiratory tract ailments such as pleurisy, it is also used to reduce pain and inflammation and ease breathing.

PSYLLIUM
Plantago psyllium
Description: The seeds contain mucilage. It has a rosette of leaves and a spike which is densely covered with purplish green flowers. The rhizome is yellow. All parts of the plant are used.

Uses: The husks are effective in the relief of constipation and also diarrhoea as the mucilage swells inside and has anti-inflammatory properties. It helps lower blood cholesterol. Externally the leaves can be applied to a wound and stop the bleeding.

RASPBERRY
Rubus idaeus
Description: The plant grows from layering and has erect stems which produce crimson berries in summer. Native to Britain, it prefers a cool climate.
Uses: The leaves made into a tea are beneficial for many women's internal problems from menstruation to childbirth. It stimulates lax bowels and relieves upset stomachs in children. It should only be used in pregnancy from the second trimester.

RHUBARB
Rheum palmatum
Description: This Asia Minor plant has long stems, red on the outside and yellow within. The leaves are palmate and rough and the plant produces a stem of white flowers in spring. This is not the cooking rhubarb.
Uses: The astringent root in small doses stops diarrhoea while in large doses it works as a laxative. Culinary rhubarb, in large amounts, also works as a laxative.

ST JOHN'S WORT
Hypericum perforatum
Description: A European herb, it grows freely up to a metre, with barren stems, pale green leaves and yellow flowers. It flowers in summer and produces black seeds with a strong smell.
Uses: Mainly used for depression and nerve pain and it can help with children's bedwetting problems when combined with cornsilk. It has been used recently in treatment of AIDS patients.

SARSAPARILLA
Smilax ornata
Description: Native to South America, it is a perennial

climber with roots up to 2 metres long. The stem has alternate leaves, prickles and no flowers or fruit to be observed.

Uses: Useful to eliminate urea and uric acid from the blood, which is needed in the case of gout and rheumatism sufferers, and occasionally psoriasis patients. It helps to improve the health of the skin. The root of the plant is the part used.

SCULLCAP
Scutellaria lateriflora
Description: Called Madweed, this North American native is a creeping perennial with downy leaves and blue and white tubular flowers.

Uses: A great nervine for spasms, excitability, epilepsy, insomnia, headache, tension, anxiety, hysteria and twitchiness. It is considered a specific for St Vitus's Dance., inducing sleep.

SENNA (see Cassia)

SENEGA
Polygala senega
Description: A North American perennial with milky sap, it grows to 24 cm, alternate leaves and produces a spike of 3cms covered in pale pink flowers. The root is the part used and is twisted and tastes like wintergreen.

Uses: Most commonly used as an expectorant to relieve bronchitis but is also used as a diuretic.

SLIPPERY ELM
Ulmus fulva
Description: This is a small tree that grows in North America with hairy rough leaves and buds covered in a yellow fluff. The inner bark of the tree is used.

Uses: Slippery elm affects the whole body, is rich in mucilage, acting rapidly by soothing the inflamed surfaces of a variety of mucous membranes and is especially beneficial for the lungs, stomach and intestines. Its soothing qualities help control diarrhoea, enteritis, colitis and gastritis, and it can be taken by either spreading the powdered bark over cereal or making it into a paste with water. Slippery elm tablets and capsules can be very convenient, depending on the condition to be treated and the age of the patient. It is as nutritious as oats and is good as a base in invalid food.

SPEARMINT
Mentha spicata
Description: A Mediterranean plant which suckers, has bright green crinkled leaves, and whorls of lilac flowers, followed by tiny brown seeds.

Uses: Used in cooking, it relieves flatulence and stomach upset. It is suitable for colic in babies and children and has diuretic properties. Mint punch, julep, vinegar, and jelly are all popular and it is said to stimulate a desire to eat meat. Mint jelly is a common accompaniment to lamb.

TEA TREE OIL
Melaleuca alternifolia
Description :A small tree, native to Australia, which was once used to make tea. The tree has a papery bark and creamy bottlebrush flowers. The oil is distilled from the leaves.

Uses: The clear oil can be used to treat skin disorders and is used for ulcers, sores, wounds, carbuncles, abscesses, fungal disorders, including tinea, and as a gargle for throat infections such as thrush. It is useful as a household disinfectant, washing floors for its refreshing smell and insect-repellant qualities, and when washing clothes.

THUJA
Thuja occidentalis
Description: A conifer tree that grows to 10 metres or more, its foliage is fragrant. The twigs are used.

Uses: Thuja stimulates the uterus and heart muscles, promotes menstruation, relieves headache, and heart pain. It can also be applied externally for warts. Thuja should not be taken during pregnancy.

THYME
Thymus vulgaris
Description: This is a common garden herb with a woody root and stems, branching from the ground up to 10 cms. The leaves are tiny and grey-green, the flowers appear in whorls and are lilac and small.

Uses: As a tea it is useful in urinary tract and digestive tract complaints, stimulating the appetite, relieving flatulence and colic, and helping relieve the symptoms of a cold. It is also used for the treatment of bronchitis and asthma.

UVA URSI (Bearberry)
Arctostaphylos uva-ursi
Description: A northern hemisphere shrub with many sprawling branches. The leaves are evergreen, flowers white with 10 brown stamens, and berries glossy red with 5 stones.

Uses: The leaves are used in bladder and kidney infections, working as an antiseptic. It has been used to treat incontinence and as a diuretic.

VALERIAN
Valeriana officinalis
Description: The conical root may take several years to develop. Stems are sent out horizontally, and at right angles, and take root. It flowers in late summer and the fruit produces one seed. Native to Britain, it thrives in damp and well-drained soil.

Uses: Valerian is a powerful muscle relaxant and a nervine. It can be used, in combination with a number of herbs, for sleeplessness, nervousness, restlessness, irritability and anxiety. Passion flower and valerian combined with a small percentage of peppermint leaves is a calming, physically soothing, mixture.

WHITE WILLOW BARK
Salix alba
Description: The bark of this European willow contains salicin. The tree is large, with rough grey bark and soft light green leaves.

Uses: Salicin was the original aspirin. It reduces inflammation and the pain of rheumatism. It is good for oral inflammations, sores and wounds, and has been used to treat digestive disorders and in herbal analgesic formulas.

WINTERGREEN
Gaultheria procumbens
Description: A small shrub, native to North America, it grows in mountainous regions and is tough with leathery leaves, single white flowers and red berries. Oil is extracted from the leaves.

Uses: Wintergreen oil treats aches and pains, including rheumatism and headache, and can reduce fever. It is readily absorbed through the skin but can cause irritation if used too often in rheumatic rubs.

References

ABRASIONS
St John Ambulance, *Australian First Aid* 1: 1990

ACNE
Ayres, S. Jnr, Mihan, R. Acne vulgaris and lipid peroxidation. New concepts in pathogenesis and treatment. *Int. J. Dermatol.* 17: 305, 1978

Department of Community Services and Health *National Dietary Survey of Adults.* 42-45, 1983

Dowining, D.T., Stewart, M.E., Wetz, P.W., Strauss, J.S. Essential fatty acids and acne. *J. Am. Acad. Dermatol.* 14: 221-5, 1986

Hubler, W.R. Unsaturated fatty acids in acne. *Arch. Dermatol.* 644-6, 1959

Kligman, A.M. et al. Oral vitamin A in acne vulgaris. *Int. J. Dermatol.* 20:278, 1981

Metal, A. Serum zinc in acne vulgaris. *Int. J. Dermatol.* 21: 481, 1982

Mihanr, A. Acne vulgaris, therapy directed at pathophysiologic defects. *Cutis.* 28: 41-2, 1981

ALLERGIES
Kaminura, M. Anti-inflammatory activity of vitamin E. *J. Vitamol.* 18 (4): 204-9, 1972

Werbach, R. *Nutritional influences on illness, A Sourcebook of Clinical Research.* 1988

ALZHEIMER'S DISEASE
Bober, M.J., Senile dementia and nutrition. Letter to the editor. *Brit. Med. J.* 288: 1234, 1984

Burns, A., Holland, T. Vitamin E deficiency. Letter to the editor. *Lancet.* 805-6, 5 April 1986

Hullin, R.P. Serum zinc in psychiatric patients. *Prog. Clin. Biol. Res.* 129: 197-206, 1983

Meydani, M. et al. Effect of vitamin E, selenium and age on lipid peroxidation events in rat cerebrum. *Nutri. Res.* 5: 1227-36, 1985

Muller, D. et al. Vitamin E in brains of patients with Alzheimer's disease and Down's syndrome. *Lancet.* 1: 1093-94, 1986

ANAEMIA
Bernat, I. Iron deficiency. *Iron Metabolism.* 215-74, Plenum Press, New York, 1983

Monsen, E.R. Ascorbic acid: an enhancing factor in iron absorption. Nutritional bioavailability of iron. *American Chemical Society.* 85-95, 1982

Natt, C.L., Machlin, L. Plasma levels of tocopherol in sickle cell anaemia subjects. *Am. J. Clin. Nutr.* 32: 1359, 1979

Pierce, L.E., Rath, C.E. Evidence for folic acid deficiency in the genesis of anaemic sickle cell crisis. *Blood.* 20: 19, 1962

ANOREXIA AND BULIMIA NERVOSA
Bryce-Smith, D., Simpson R.I.D. Anorexia, depression and zinc deficiency. *Lancet.* 2: 1162, 1984

Langan, S.M., Farrell, P.M. *Am. J. Clin. Nutr.* 41: 1054-60, 1985

Safai-Kutti, S., Kutte, J. Zinc and anorexia nervosa. *Ann. Int. Med.* 100: 317-18, 1984

ARTHRITIS
British Herbal Medicine Association *British Herbal Pharmacopoeia.* West Yorkshire, 1983

Kremer, J.M. Effects of manipulation of dietary fatty acids on clinical manifestations of rheumatoid arthritis. *Lancet.* 1: 184-7, 1985

Horrobin, D.F. The importance of gamma-linolenic acid and prostoglandin E in human nutrition and medicine. *J. Holistic Med.* 3: 118-139, 1981

General practitioner research group. Calcium pantothenate in arthritic conditions. *Practitioner.* 224: 208-11, 1980

ASTHMA
British Herbal Medicine Association *British Herbal Pharmacopoeia.* West Yorkshire, 1983

Horrobin, D.F. Omega-6, Essential fatty acids, *Pathophysiology and Roles in Clinical Medicine.* 1990

Pizzorno, J. and Murray, M. A textbook of natural medicine. John Bastyr College Publications, 1987

Kay, A.B., Mediators of hypersensitivity and inflammatory cells in the pathogenesis of bronchial asthma. *Euro J Resp Dis Suppl.* 129: 1-45, 1983

Lindahl, O., Lindwall L. et al. Vegan diet regimen with reduced medication in the treatment of bronchial asthma. *J Asthma.* 22: 45-55, 1985

Felter, H. *The eclectic materia medica. Pharmacology and therapeutics.* Eclectic Med. Pub. Portland, Or., 1983

Dorsch, W. et al. Antiasthmatic effects of onion extracts. Detection of benzyl and other isothiocyanates in mustard oils as antiasthmatic compounds of plant origin. *Euro J Pharmacol.* 107: 17 - 24, 1985

Mohsenin, V. et al Effect of ascorbic acid on response to methacholine challenge in asthmatic subjects. *Am. Rev. Respir. Dis.* 127: 143-7, 1983

Lee, T.H., Arm, J.P. Prospects for modifying the allergic response by fish oil diets. *Clin. Allergy.* 16(2): 89-100, 1986

Schacter, E.N., Schlesinger, A. The attenuation of exercise-induced bronchospasm by ascorbic acid. *Ann. Allergy.* 49: 146-50, 1982

Mink, K.A., Dick, E.C., et al. Amelioration of rhinovirus colds by vitamin C (ascorbic acid) supplementation. *Symposium of Med.Virology.* Calif., 12 Nov 1987

Australian Medical Association. *Guide to medicines and drugs* . 1990

BITES AND STINGS
St John Ambulance *Australian First Aid.* 1: 180-199, 1990

BLOOD PRESSURE IN PREGNANCY
O'Brien, P.M.S. et al. The effect of dietary supplementation with linoleic acid and linolenic acid on the pressor response to angiotensin 11, A possible role in pregnancy-induced hypertension? *Brit. J. Clin. Pharmacol.* 19(3): 335-42, 1985

BRONCHITIS
Mills, S. *The Dictionary of Modern Herbalism.* Lothian, Sydney, 1985

CANCER
Belman, S. Onion and garlic oil inhibit tumor growth. *Carcginogenesis.* 4 (8): 1063-5, 1983

Carper, J. Fish oil and cancer. *The Courier Mail*, 6 June 1990

Clark, L.C. and Combs, Selenium compounds and the prevention of cancer. Research needs and public implications. *J. Nutr.* 166: 170-176, 1986

Florence, T.M., *T*he role of free radicals in cancer and ageing, in trace elements, micronutrients and free radicals. Humana Press, New York 1990

Florence, T.M., Cancer and ageing, the free radical connection. *Chem. Australia.* 50: 166-174, 1983

Gey, K.F., Brubacher, G.B., and Stahelin, H.B., Plasma levels of antioxidant vitamins in relation to heart diseases and cancer. *Amer. J. Clin. Nutr.* 45,: 1363-1377, 1987

Graham, S. et. al. Dietary factors in the epidemiology of cancer of the larynx. *Am. J. Epid.* 113 (6): 675-80, 1981

Horrobin, D. *Med. Hypotheses.* 6, 469-86, 1980

Menkes, M.S., et al. Serum beta carotene, vitamins A and E, selenium and the risk of lung cancer. *New Engl. J.*

Med. 315: 1250, 1986
    Modan, B. et. al. *J. National Cancer Instit.* 55: 15-18, 1975
    National Academy of Sciences. *Nutrition, Diet and Cancer.* 1982
    Stich, H.F., et al. A pilot beta-carotene intervention trial using smokeless tobacco. *Int. J. Cancer* 36: 321, 1985

COLD SORES (HERPES SIMPLEX)
    Fitzherbert, J. Genital herpes and zinc. *Med. J. Aust.* 1: 399, 1979
    Griffith, R., Norins, A. A multicentred study of lysine therapy in herpes simplex infection. *Dermatol* . 156: 257-67, 1978
    Terazhealmy, G., Bottomley, W. and Pellu, G. The use of water soluble bioflavonoid - ascorbic acid complex in the treatment of recurrent herpes labialis. *Oral Surg.* 45: 56-62, 1978

DIABETES MELLITUS
    Peifer, J.J., Holman, R.T. Essential fatty acid, diabetes and cholesterol *Arch. Biochem. Bio. Phys.* 57: 520-1, 1965
    Potter, J. Glucose metabolism in glucose tolerant older people during chromium supplementation. *Metabolism* 34: 199-204, 1985
    Som, S. Ascorbic acid metabolism in diabetes mellitus. *Metabolism* 30 (6): 572-7, 1981
    Tarui, S. Studies of zinc metabolism. Effect of the diabetic state on zinc metabolism. A clinical aspect. *Endocrin.* (Japan) 10: 9-15, 1963

EPILEPSY
    Crayton, J.W. Epilepsy precipitated by food sensitivity. Report of a case with double-blind placebo-controlled assessment. *Clin. Electroencephalo.* 2 (4): 192-8, 1981
    Mantovani, J. Effects of taurine on seizures and growth hormone release in epileptic patients. *Arch. Neuro.* 35: 1979

Nakazawa. M. High dose vitamin B6 therapy in infantile spasms. The effects and adverse reactions. *Brain and Development* 5(2): 193, 1983

Roach, E.S., Carlin, L.N., N-dimethylglycine for epilepsy (letter to ed.) *N. Eng. Med. J.* 307: 1081-82, 1982

Shoji, Y. Serum magnesium and zinc in epileptic children. *Brain and Dev.* 5 (2): 200, 1983

EYESIGHT
Sala, D. Effect of anthocyanosides on visual performance at low illumination. *Minerva Oftamol* 21: 283-5, 1979

Underwood, B. Vitamin A in animal and human nutrition in the retina. Academic Press, 1984

FISH AND FISH LIVER OILS
Das, U.N. Antibiotic-like action of essential fatty acids. *Can. Med. Assoc. J.* 132: 1350, 1985

Kremer, J.M. Effects of manipulation of dietary fatty acids on clinical manifestation of rheumatiod arthritis. *Lancet* 1: 184-7, 1985

Kirschmann, J. Nutrition Search Inc. *Nut. Almanac* 1979

Vitamin A in Breast Milk,*Myles Textbook for Midwives.* 492, 1990

Sanders, T.B.A., Vickers, A.P. et al. Effect on blood lipids and haemostasis of a supplement of cod liver oil, rich in eicosapentaenoic and docosahexaenoic acids, in healthy young men. *Clin. Sci.* 61: 317-24, 1981

Saynor, R. The long term effect of dietary supplementation with fish lipid concentrate on serum lipids, bleeding time, platelets and angina. *Atherosclerosis* 50,:3-10, 1984

Wood, D.A. Linoleic and eicosapentaenoic acids in adipose tissue and platelets and risk of coronary heart disease. *Lancet.* 1:176-82, 1987

HEADACHES
British Herbal Pharmacopoeia. West Yorkshire, 1983

Greden, J.F. Caffeine withdrawal headache, A clinical profile. *Psychosomatics* 21: 411-18, 1980

Shirlow, M.J., Mathers, C.D. A study of caffeine consumption and symptom, indigestion, palpitation, tremor, headache and insomnia *Int. J. Epidemiol* 14(2): 239-48, 1985

HEART DISEASE
Bordia, A.K., Verma, S.K. Garlic found to regress atherosclerosis in rabbits. *Artery* 7: 428, 1980

Burch, G.E., Giles, T.D. The importance of magnesium deficiency in cardiovascular disease. *Lancet* 1: 1044-6, 1977

Lady Cilento You don't have to live with ailing heart and blood vessels. 1977

Erst, E. Garlic and blood lipids. *British Med. J.* 291: 139, 1985

Herold, P.M. Fish oil consumption and decreased risk of cardio-vascular disease; a comparison of findings from animal and human feeding. *Trials Am. Nut. J.* 43: 566-98, 1986

Herman, W.J. The effect of tocopherol on high-density lipoprotein cholesterol, a clinical observation. *Am. J. Clin. Path.* 72: 848-52, 1979

HEPATITIS
Campbell, R.E., Pruitt, F.W. Vitamin B12 in the treatment of viral hepatitis. *Am. J. Med. Sci.* 224: 252, 1952

HORMONE REPLACEMENT THERAPY
Harju, E. et al. High incidence of low serum vitamin D concentration in patients with hip fracture. *Arch. Orthoped, and Trauma Surg.* 103(6): 408-16, 1985

Nordian, B.E. et al. A prospective trial of the effect of vitamin D supplementation on metacarpal bone loss in elderly women. *Am. J. Clin. Nutr.* 42(3): 470-74, 1985

Pizzorno, J. , Murray, M. *A textbook of natural medicine.* John Bastyr College Publications, 1987

HYPOGLYCAEMIA
Anderson, R.A. Chromium supplementation of humans with hypoglycaemia. *Fed. Proc.* 43: 471, 1984

Curry, D.L. Magnesium modulation of glucose induced insulin secretion by the perfused rat pancreas *Endocrinology* 101: 203, 1977

Sanders, L.R. Refined carbohydrate as a contributing factor in reactive hypoglycaemia. *Southern Med. J.* 75: 1072, 1982

IMMUNE SYSTEM
Bland, J.S. *Chronic Infections and Immune Function.* 1988

Cathcart, R.F. Vitamin C in the treatment of Acquired Immune Deficiency Syndrome (AIDS). *Med. Hypotheses* 14: 423-33, 1984

Cavallito, C.J., Bailey, J.H. Allicin, the antibacterial principle of *Allium sativum*.Isolation, physical properties and antibacterial action. *J. Am. Chem. Soc.* 66: 1950-51, 1944

Elamin, I., Elnim Syed, A., Abdel, G., Mossa, J. The antimicrobial activity of garlic and onion extracts. *Pharmazie* 38: 747, 1983

Huddleson, I.F., Dufrain, J., Barrons, K.C., Geifel, M. Anti-bacterial substances in plants. *J. Am. Vet. Med. Assoc.* 105: 394-7, 1944

Keith, M.D., Pelletier, O. Ascorbic acid concentration in leukocytes and selected organs of guinea pigs in response to the increasing ascorbic acid intake. *Am. J. Clin. Nut.* 27: 368, 1974

Mose, J. Effect of Echinacin on Phagocytosis and Natural Killer Cells. *Med. Welt.* 34: 1423-33, 1984

Pizzorno. J, and Murray, M. *Textbook of Natural Medicine*, John Bastyr Publications,1985

Takahashi,I. Nakanishi, S. Hypericin and pseudohypericin specifically inhibit protein kinase C; Possible relation to their antiretroviral activity. *Biochem. Biophysical Res, Comm.* 165 (3): 1207-12, 1989

Vahera, S.B., Rizwan, M., Khan, J.A. Medical Uses of Common Indian Vegetables. *Planta Med.* 23: 381-93, 1973

Wagner, V., Proksch, A., Riess-Maurer, I.

Immunostimulating Polysaccharides (heteroglycans) of Higher Plants. Preliminary Communications *Arzneim Forsch* 34, 659-60, 1984

Tsai, Y., Cole, L.L., Davis, L.E., Lockwood, S. J., Simmons, V.,Wild, G.C. Antiviral properties of garlic. In vitro effects of influenza B, herpes simplex and coxsackie viruses. *Plant Medica* 460: Oct. 1985

MEMORY

Dysken, M.A. Review of recent clinical trials in the treatment of Alzheimer's Dementia. *Psychiatric Annals* 17 (3): 178, 1987

Hindmarch, I. The psychopharmacological effects of *Ginkgo biloba* extract in normal healthy volunteers. *Int. J. Clin. Pharmacol. Res.* 4: 39-43, 1984

King, R.G. Do raised aluminium levels in Alzheimer's Dementia cause cholinergic neuronal deficits? *Med. Hypoth.* 14: 301-6, 1984

Muller, D. Vitamin E in brains of patients with Alzheimer's Disease and Down's Syndrome. *Lancet* 1: 1093-4, 1986

MENOPAUSE

British Herbal Pharmacopoeia West Yorkshire, 1983

Duke, J.A., Ayensu, E.S. *Medicinal Plants of China* Reference Publication, 1985

Finkler, R.S. The effects of vitamin E in the menopause *J. Clin. Endocrin. Metabol.* 9: 89-94, 1949

Smith, C.J. Non-hormonal control of vaso-motor flushing in menopausal patients. *Chicago Med.* 7 March 1964

MENSTRUATION

Bettini, V. Effects of Vaccinium myrtillus anthocyanosides on vascular smooth muscle. *Fitoterapia* 55: 265-72, 1984

Butler, E.B., McKnight, E. Vitamin E in the treatment of

primary dysmenorrhoea *Lancet* 1,: 1844-47, 1955

Stuart, M.(ed) *The Encyclopaedia of Herbs and Herbalism.* Orbis Publishing, Bristol, 1979

OSTEOPOROSIS

Barzel, U.S. Acid loading and osteoporosis. *J. Am. Geriatrics Soc.* Sept. 1982

Draper, H.H., Scythes, C.A. Calcium, phosphorous and osteoporosis *Fed. Proc.* 40(9): 2434-38, 1981

Hollingbery, P.W. Effect of dietary caffeine and aspirin on urinary calcium and hydroxyproline excretion in pre- and menopausal women. *Fed. Proc.* 44: 1149, 1985

Worthington-Roberts, B. *Contemporary Developments in Nutrition* St Lewis, M.O., C.V., Mosby Co., 1981

PARKINSONS DISEASE

Pincus J.H., Barry K *Arch. Neurol.* March, 1987

Mena I., Manganese, I., Bronner F, et al. *Disorders of mineral metabolism.* New York, Academic Press, 1981

Long, B., James W. *Prescription Drugs.* N.Y., Harper & Row, 1980

Bianchine, J.R. *New Eng J. Med.* 295: 814, 1976

Boissier, J.R. General pharmacology of ergot alkaloids. *Pharmacology.* 16: Suppl. 1, 12, 1978

British Herbal Pharmacopoeia. West Yorkshire, 1983

Critchley, E.M. Evening primrose oil (efamol) in Parkinson's and other tremors, *Clinical Use of Essential Fatty Acids.* Montreal, Eden Press, 205-8, 1982

Heller, B. et al. Therapeutic action of D-phenylalinine in Parkinson's disease, *Arzneim-Forsch* 26: 577-79, 1976

Merck Manual (fifteenth edition) 1421-1424, 1987

Pfeiffer, C.C. *Mental and elemental nutrients.* Conn., Keats Pub Co. 1975

Sacks, W. *Lancet* March, 1975

Smythies, J.R. et al, Treatment of Parkinson's disease. *South Med.* 77: 1577, 1984

PREGNANCY

Gold, S., Sherry, L. Hyperactivity, learning disabilities and alcohol. *J. Learning Disabilities* 17(1): 3-6, 1984

Laurence, K.M. Double-blind randomized controlled trial of folate treatment before conception to prevent recurrence of neural tube defects. *Brit. Med. J.* 282: 1509, 1981

Mowrey, R. *Scientific Validation of Herbal Medicine.* Keats Publishing, Connecticut, 1986

O'Brien, P.M.S. The effect of dietary supplementation with linoleic acid and linolenic acid on the pressor response to angotensin 11. A possible role in pregnancy-induced hypertension. *British J. Clin. Pharmacol.* 19(3): 335-42, 1985

Smitheus, R.W. Apparent prevention of neural tube defects by periconceptional vitamin supplementation. *Arch. Dis. Childhood* 56: 911, 1981

Sutton, R.V. Vitamin E in habitual abortion. *Brit. Med. J.* 4 Oct. 1958

Tolarovam, M. Periconceptional supplementation with vitamins and folic acid to prevent recurrence of cleft lip. *Lancet* 2: 217, 1982

VITAMIN A AND PREGNANCY

Das, U.N. Antibiotic-like action of essential fatty acids. *Can. Med. Assoc. J.* 132:1350. 1985.

Kirschmann J. Nutrition Search, Inc. *Nutritional Almanac* (rev. ed) 1979

Kremer, J.M. et al. Effects of manipulation of dietary fatty acids on clinical manifestations of rheumatoid arthritis. *Lancet* 1: 184-7, 1985

Vitamin A in breast milk.*Myles Textbook For Midwives,* 492, 1990

Sanders,T.B.A., Vickers, A.P. et al. Effect on blood lipids and haemostasis of a supplement of cod liver oil, rich in eicosapentaenoic and docosahexaenoic acids, in healthy young men. *Clin. Sci.* 61: 317-24 (1981)

Saynor, R. et al. The long-term effect of dietary supplementation with fish lipid concentrate on serum lipids, bleed-

ing time, platelets and angina. *Atherosclerosis* 50: 3-10, 1984
    Wood, D.A. et al. Linoleic and eicosapentaenoic acids in adipose tissue and platelets and risk of coronary heart disease. *Lancet* 1:176-82, 1987

PMT
    Barr, W. Pyridoxine supplements in the premenstrual syndrome. *Practitioner* 228: 425-7, 1984
    Horrobin, D.F. The role of essential fatty acids and prostaglandins in the premenstrual syndrome. *J. Reprod. Med.* 28 (7): 465-68, 1983
    Piesse, J.W. Nutritional factors in the premenstrual syndrome. *Int. Clin. Nutr. Rev.* 4: 54-81, 1984

TINNITUS
    British Herbal Pharmacopoeia West Yorkshire, 1983
    Browning, G.G. Blood viscosity as a factor in sensorineural hearing impairment. *Lancet* 1,: 121-23, 1986
    Dolev, E. Is magnesium depletion the reason for ototoxicity caused by aminoglycosides? *Med. Hypotheses* 10(4): 353-58, 1983
    Vorberg, G. *Ginkgo biloba* extract (GBE), A long term study of chronic cerebral insufficiency in geriatric patients. *Clinical Trials J.* 22: 149-57, 1985

VARICOSE VEINS
    Fuji, T. The clinical effects of vitamin E on purpuras due to vascular defects. *J. Vitaminology* 18, 125-30, 1972
    Shapiro, S. Spitzer, J.M. The use of cepevit (ascorbic acid plus 'P' factors) in drug-induced hypoprothrombinemia. *Angiology* 5: 64-71, 1954

VITAMIN A
    Australian Medical Association, *Guide To Medicines & Drugs.* 382, 1990
    Balch, J.F. , Balch, P.A. *Prescription for Nutritional Healing.* 1990

INDEX

abrasions 34, 83, 155
abscesses 157
acidophilus 56-7, 71, 78, 88, 114
Acne vulgaris 35, 101, 143
Addison's disease 152
ageing 36-39
agrimony 89
Agropyrum repens 142
AIDS 107, 155
alcohol 5, 41, 121, 123, 129,
147, 152
alfalfa (Lucerne) 49, 136
allergies 39, 51-2, 79, 80,
85, 88, 103,119
Allium sativum 146
Aloe spp 136
Aloe vera 62, 70-1, 133, 136
aluminium 45
Alzheimer's disease 43-5
amines 39, 40, 42, 64
anaemia 46, 143
anal fissures 47
Anethum graveoluens 143
Angelica sinensis 143
angina 111
aniseed 27, 41, 136
Anorexia nervosa 48, 147
antibiotics 71, 91, 114, 122,
130-1, 142
antioxidants 37, 39, 44-5, 65,
94-5, 112
anxiety 149, 154, 158, 153,
156
Apgar scale 31
Apium graveolens 140
apricot kernel oil 59
Arctium lappa 139
Arctostaphylos uva-ursi 158
arnica 69
arthritis 49-50, 97-8, 111, 122, 149
Asclepias tuberosa 154
asthma 51-5, 85, 99, 124,
144-5, 149, 158
athlete's foot 55-6
Avena sativa 153
barberry 137
barley water 84

bayberry 137
bearberry 84
beclomethasone (becotide) 52, 54
bedwetting 57, 141, 155
belladonna 124
Berberis vulgaris 137
beta-carotene 37, 44, 64-5,
94-5, 109-110, 136
Betonica officinalis 137
betony 137
bicarbonate of soda 60, 72, 79
bifidus 56-7, 71, 78, 88, 114
bioflavonoids 43, 47, 49, 54,
69, 118
birthmarks 59
bites and stings 60-1, 136,143, 153
black cohosh 137, 143
bladder 142, 149, 150, 158
blisters 61-62
blueberry (bilberry) 95
blood poisoning 62-63
blood pressure 16, 144-5, 147, 149
boils 63, 143-4, 146
boldo 84, 101, 138
breast cancer 64, 110
breastfeeding 10, 25
  calcium requirements 27
  colostrum 26
  cow's milk compared 29
  'let down' reflex 26
  milk production 27, 152
  nutrition 27, 146
  position 26
  preparation 2
  vitamins 26
breast self-examination 66-7
brewer's yeast 27, 87, 131
bronchitis 57, 68, 74, 144,
146-7, 150-1, 154, 156, 158
bruises 69, 136, 144, 153
buchu 84
buckthorn 138
bulimia 48
burdock 36, 63, 85, 139
burns 61-62, 70, 136,141,
144, 153
caffeine 94, 123, 151
calcium 14, 27-8, 103-5,

121, 123, 126, 136
calendula 62, 83
camphor 15, 82, 139
cancer 64-6, 112
candidiasis (thrush) 71, 109,
118, 142, 147, 157
cape aloes 81
Capsicum minimum 140
carbohydrates 94, 106, 118-19
cardamon 41
cardiovascular disease 94, 97,
107, 111, 120, 149, 151-3
carrageen 150
Cascara sagrada 81, 139
Cassia senna 140
cataracts 94, 111
cayenne 41, 140
celery 84, 140
celery seed 50
cervix 21, 31
chamomile 25
charcoal 57, 114
chillies 135
chickenpox 72
chickweed 85-6, 140
childbirth 15, 155
chlorophyll 57
choking 73-4
cholesterol 145, 147-8,
153, 155
Chondrus crispus 150
chromium 107
cigarette smoking 6, 65,
74-5, 121, 123
Cimicifuga racemosa 137
Cinnamomum camphora 139
cinnamon 41
citronella 60
cloves 41, 141
Cochlearia amoracia 150
cod liver oil 29, 36, 50, 55,
62, 68-9, 75-6, 89, 91, 96,
99, 104-5, 128, 130
Cola nitida 151
cold and flu 75-76, 144-5, 150, 158
cold sores 77-78, 108
colic 79, 114, 136, 141, 143,
154, 157-8

colitis 136, 156
colostrum 26, 28
comfrey 34, 59, 141
conception 1-2
concussion 79
conjunctivitis 80, 145
constipation 57, 80-81, 142,
14ᵈ 154-5
contractions 21, 24, 31
corn silk 84 , 141, 155
corn starch 86
cornflour 56, 71-2, 117
couch grass 84, 141
cow's milk 15, 28-9, 39, 50,
79, 86, 88
cramps 136
cranesbill 142
Crataegus officinale 149
croup 82
crying 82
cuts 83
Cynara scolymus 148
cystitis 83, 144
cytotoxic blood test 40
dandelion 3, 4, 85, 101, 102,
142
Datura stramonium 124
deadly nightshade 124
depression 151, 153
dermatitis 85, 101
diabetes 86-7, 95, 106, 152
diarrhoea 71, 81, 87-8, 136,
142, 144, 154-6
digestion 136, 146-7, 150,
158-9
digestive bitters 57
dill 79, 103, 143, 146
diuretic 141-2, 149-50,
156-8
dizziness 16, 89
dong quai 104-5, 116, 143
dyslexia 90
earache 91
Echinacea angustifolia 36,
63-4, 68,143, 73, 76-8, 80,
83, 88-9, 91, 109, 112-3,
130, 132-4
eclampsia 17

eczema 85-6, 145
egg 8
elder flower 96, 144
embryo 17, 31
emergency childbirth 23-4
epilepsy 92-4, 151, 154, 156
Equisetum arvense 150
ergot of rye 124-125
Eucalyptus globulus 15, 68, 76, 82, 129, 144
Eugenia carophyllata 141
Euphorbia hirta 54-5, 68, 82, 145
Euphrasia officinalis 145
evening primrose oil 14, 38-9, 85-6, 104-5, 116, 126, 145
exercise 11-13, 20, 38, 104
eyebright 80, 145
eyes and eyesight 94, 144-5, 148
fallopian tubes 31
false labour 21
fats 119-20
fennel 27, 146
fenugreek 27, 146
fetus 4-5, 17, 18-20, 32
fever 62, 68, 72-3, 83, 88, 91, 96-97, 100-101, 129, 146
feverfew 146
fish oil 49-50, 64-5, 95, 97-9, 104
fits 17
flatulence 141, 146, 157-8
Foeniculum vulgare 27-8, 146
folic acid 8, 46-7, 123
food additives 40
free radicals 37, 44, 94, 111
Friar's balsam 28
Fucus vesiculosus 151
Galega officinalis 27
gall bladder 150
garlic 45, 54, 65, 68, 72, 76, 88-9, 91-2, 108-9, 112,113, 122, 128, 130, 134, 146
gastric disorders 136, 154
gastric reflux 45
Gaultheria procumbens 159
gentian 147
Gentiana lutea 147
Geranium maculatum 142
German measles (rubella) 99

ginger 15, 41, 117
Ginkgo biloba 44-5, 90
ginsana 44-5
ginseng 44, 147
glaucoma 95
globe artichoke 148
Glycyrrhiza glabra 152
goat's milk 39, 71, 79, 88
goat's rue 27
golden seal 62, 80, 83, 113, 132, 148
gout 149, 156
Grindelia camporum 54-5, 69, 148
gripe water 79
groin 102
Guaiacum officinale 50, 149
haemorrhoids 142, 153
halitosis (bad breath) 57
hawthorn 149, 151
headache 16, 100, 146, 151, 154, 156, 159
heart disease 74, 122
heartburn 45
hepatitis 100-102, 152
hernia 102
hiccups 102-103, 136
hives (urticaria) 103
home birth 22-5
honey 41
hops 75, 93, 105, 149
horehound 68, 149
hormones 15, 32, 35, 38, 101, 122
Hormone Replacement Therapy 103-105
horseradish 89, 92, 128, 150
horsetail 150
Humulus lupulus 149
Hydrastis canadensis 148
hyperactivity 105
Hypericum perforatum 155
hypoglycaemia 106-107
hypothermia 107
immune system 63, 76, 78, 94, 96, 107,110, 130, 132, 134
impetigo 112-113
indigestion 113, 149, 151
insomnia 136, 149, 156, 158
iodine 151

irish moss 150
iron 26, 46, 53, 89, 101, 121, 136
iron phosphate 63, 77
jaundice 148, 150
juniper 84-5, 151
Juniperus communis 151
kelp 151
kidneys 3, 6, 7, 16, 84, 111,
142, 150, 152-3, 158
kola 151
Lactobacillus acidophilus 71
lactose 29, 30, 88
lanolin (wool fat) 28, 47, 86
laxative 152, 155
lecithin 126
lice 115
lime flowers 151
liquor amnii 21
liquorice 40, 54, 68-9, 152
liver 16, 17, 62, 142, 147-8, 152
lobelia 124
lysine 78
mace 41
magnesium phosphate 90, 107, 123,
131
manganese 126
Marrubium vulgare 149
marshmallow 63, 69, 84
mastectomy 66
Medico sativa 136
Melaleuca alternifolia 157
menopause 66, 122-3, 143, 153
menstruation 115-116, 143, 145-7,
148-50, 155
Mentha piperita 154
Mentha spicata 157
menthol 68, 82
migraine 40, 100, 151
milk thistle 101, 152
minerals 121- 122
mint 41
miscarriage 14, 74
mistletoe 151
molasses 8
monosodium glutamate 43
morning sickness 15
motion sickness 117, 147
mullein 68, 152

Myrica cerifera 137
nappy rash 117, 153
nasal congestion 15
nasal spray formula 92, 129
neural tube defects 46
neuralgia 150
night vision 95
nipples, cracked 28
nitrosamines 64
nosebleed 118
Nursing Mothers' Association 26
nutrition 1, 5, 27, 118-119
oats 153
oestrogen 103-4
Olea europaea 153
olive oil 153
Oenothera biennis 145
oregano 153
Origanum vulgare 153
osteoporosis 103-4, 122-3
palpitations 151
Panax ginseng 147
pantothenic acid 50
paprika 41
paraffin 47
Parkinson's disease 123-6
Passiflora incarnata 105
passion flower 75, 93, 125, 154, 158
peppermint 25, 57, 79, 96,
114-115, 117, 146, 154
Peumus boldus 138
phosphorus 136
Pimpinella anisum 136
pine coal tar 85-6
placenta 3, 4, 17, 22, 25-6
Plantago psyllium 154
pleurisy root 68, 154
PMT (see Premenstrual
Tension)
Polygala senega 156
post-viral syndrome 112
potassium chloride 63, 77
potassium metabisulphite 40
potassium phosphate 90, 131
prednisone 152
pregnancy 1-2, 17-20, 151-2, 155, 157
  afterbirth 31
    amniotic fluid 4, 31

breaking of waters 21
cervix, dilation 21
contractions 21
development of baby 17-20
drugs and medication 5
exercise 11-13, 20
false labour 21
fluid retention 3
glossary of terms 31
nutrition 1, 5, 46
rubella 99
shortness of breath 16
'show' at onset of labour 21
smoking 6
tiredness 2
urinary tract 84
weight gain 4
premenstrual tension 116, 130
protein 29, 30, 49, 51, 119-20, 122, 125
psoriasis 156
pumpkin 8
purple coneflower 143
Radio-Allergo Sorbent Test 40
Rhamnus catharticus 138
Rhamnus purshiana 139
raspberry 15, 16, 103
red clover 36, 85
respiratory complaints 152-4
Reye's syndrome 73, 97
Rheum palmatum 155
rheumatism 149
rhubarb 155
ringworm 127
Rubus idaeus 155
saccharin 66
sage 41
St Anthony's Fire 124
St John's wort 58, 155
salicylates 39, 40-1, 53, 105
Salix alba 158
Sambucus nigra 144
sarsaparilla 36, 85, 155
scullcap 75, 93, 105, 125, 156
Scutellaria lateriflora 156
sedative 153
selenium 39, 44, 65
senega 69, 156
senile dementia 43-4

senna 81, 140
septicaemia 62-63, 143
sesame seeds 8
sexual potency 148
shock 127-8
sialorrhea 124
silica 63
Silybum marianum 101, 152
sinusitis 57, 108, 128, 144,
145-6, 148, 150
slippery elm 45, 63, 69, 89,
114-15, 156
Smilax ornata 155
snoring 129
sodium phosphate 58
sodium sulphate 36, 40, 102
soy beans 122
soy milk 15, 30, 39, 51, 79, 88
spearmint 157
spirulina 49
staphylococcus 112
Stellaria media 140
Still's disease 49
stop itch formula 72, 99
streptococcus 112
stress 130-132
sty 132-133
sucrose 30
sulphite 39, 40
sunburn 133
sunflower seeds 78
swelling feet, legs 16
Symphytum officinale 141
tartrazine 51
Taraxacum officinale 142
tea tree oil 35-6, 52, 56, 59, 60, 62, 68,
71, 83, 113-15, 117-18, 127, 157
temperature, 16, 49, 73
thrush (see candidiasis)
Thuja occidentalis 134, 157
thyme 36, 55, 157
Thymus vulgaris 158
thyroid 151
Tilia cordata 151
tinea 157
tinnitus 89
tonsillitis 129-30
toothache 141

toxaemia (pre-eclampsia) 16
Trigonella foenum-graecum 27, 146
typhoid 147
ulcers 45, 114, 136, 142, 144
Ulmus fulva 156
umbilical cord 22, 24-5, 32
uterus 157
Uva ursi 158
Vaccinium myrtillus 138
valerian 75, 100, 105, 125, 158
Valeriana officinalis 158
vaporiser liquid 68, 76, 82
ventolin (Salbutamol) 52-3
Verbascum thapsus 152
vertigo 89
vinegar 61
vitamins, general 121-2, 131
vitamin A 7, 8, 9, 34-5, 37, 44, 55, 65,
68, 75-6, 85-6, 95, 97,101, 109-110, 128,
134
vitamin B 46, 50, 78, 101-2, 104, 116
 stress, effect 130-132
  B1 (thiamin) 126
  B6 (pyridoxine) 4, 15, 43, 60, 75
  caution using B6 125-6
  B12 46, 53, 101, 143
vitamin C 26-7, 34, 37, 39, 42,
44, 46-7, 50, 53-4, 56, 59, 60,
62, 65, 68, 70,73, 75-6, 78,
82, 87, 89, 91, 94-5, 97,
103, 110-111, 113, 118,
130, 132-4, 136
vitamin D 7, 26, 97, 101, 105, 123, 136
vitamin E (tocopherol) 7, 14,
 34-37, 39, 43-4, 59, 65,
70-1, 75, 83, 87, 93-5,
110-12, 133-4, 136, 143
vitamin K 7, 101, 136
varicose veins 152
vitex agnus-castus 116, 143
warts 134, 145, 153, 157
water 119
weight loss 134
wheat germ 8
white willow bark 50, 91, 100, 158
wintergreen oil 68, 82, 159
witch hazel 47
Woolwich nipple shield 28

yarrow 96
yellow dock 36
yoghurt 71, 78, 114, 118
Zea mays 84, 141
zinc 8, 34-5, 39, 44, 48, 56,
65, 70, 78, 85-7, 102, 117, 121, 133
zinc cream 86, 103
zinc oxide 71-2, 116
Zingiber officinale 147